THINKING
HANDS

Thinking Hands

The Little Book
on the Handiwork
of Canadian Osteopathic Medical
and Manual Practitioners
in Ousting Pain and Discomfort

by Atily Gunaratne
with John Yuen

Thinking Hands: The Little Book on the Handiwork of Canadian Osteopathic Medical and Manual Practitioners in Ousting Pain and Discomfort.

ISBN-13: 978-0-9940913-0-7
First edition.

Cover design by Elina Mer, Merstudio, elina.mer@gmail.com
Interior design by Woven Red Author Services, www.WovenRed.ca

Published by Osteopathic Health Centre
Suite 105
7777 Kipling Ave.
Vaughan, ON L4L 2Z3
905-266-2199
Fax: 905-266-2155
Email: info@thinkinghands.ca
Website: www.thinkinghands.ca

Library and Archives Canada Cataloguing in Publication.

Thinking Hands
Atily Gunaratne, John Yuen.

OSTEOPATHY: WHAT IT IS

Osteopathy is a distinctive health care system and whole-person philosophy of medicine that is devoted to treating disease and promoting health by accessing the body's natural abilities to self-heal or creatively compensate.

The art and science of osteopathy recognizes that disturbances of anatomic structure and physiologic function are interrelated and are treated utilizing a patient-specific dynamic.

Osteopathic Manipulative Treatment (OMT) is the unique form of hands-on healing or manual medicine utilized by an osteopath.

The goal of osteopathic treatment is to make every effort to discover the causes of disease and pain by restoring balance and removing the obstructions to healing thus encouraging an inherent therapeutic process.

Osteopathic manipulation uses a comprehensive and anatomically specific approach to diagnosis and treatment by restoring a healthy relationship between all of the organ systems, including the musculoskeletal system.

**—Steve Paulus, DO, Vermont, U.S.A.,
in a 2015 forthcoming article**

DEDICATION

This book is dedicated to the thousands of osteopathic practitioners, both medical and manual, and students of osteopathy who have helped and are helping millions of Canadians enjoy a more vibrant lifestyle.

ACKNOWLEDGEMENTS

An effort to pull together many strands of information and to make it comprehensible to ordinary folks would not have been possible without the insights and viewpoints of a great number of people.

Thanks to all who have been so gracious to engage with us in a dialogue about osteopathy!

First, there were those patients from chapters 2 through 14 who revealed very personal—medical, psychological, emotional and social—details of their lives.

Second, there were the busy officials who provided intelligent and coherent commentaries on the state of osteopathy in Canada. They include the spokespersons for medical regulatory authorities, national and provincial associations of both osteopathic medical and manual practitioners, political science experts from coast-to-coast whose research interests include lobbying and interest group dynamics, and doctors of osteopathic medicine and osteopathic manual practitioners.

Special thanks to Dr. Ted Findlay, past president of the Canadian Osteopathic Association; Gail Abernethy, president of the Canadian Federation of Osteopaths; and Chantale Bertrand, a Toronto-based osteopathic manual practitioner and a past board member of the Ostéopathie Québec (formerly the Association des Ostéopathes du Québec).

Third, the library assistants in the Toronto Public Library system, the City of Pickering Library, and the university library system, especially the University of Toronto Library in Mississauga, will never be forgotten for providing yeoman service in identifying and fetching documents towards the cause.

Fourth, to book and journal article authors and newspapers, such as *The Toronto Star* and *The Globe and Mail*, in particular, the author expresses his gratitude for the use of their records of past events related to osteopathy in Canada.

Fifth, I wish to thank those, who, hopefully with beverages at hand, spent many hours reading the book from cover to cover to uncover things that were written that didn't make sense—and importantly, flagged them. Their suggestions on how to make the book more readable and appealing helped enormously. Special thanks and appreciation to Paul Braithwaite, Bob Fanous, Ginette Kanyo, John Stefaniak, Roger Smithies, Wendy Terry, Mike Tweedle and the Rev. Daniel L. Graves, most of whom provided reviews of the book (please see the outside back cover).

Sixth, as a large portion of the book will appeal to students of osteopathy and practitioners of osteopathy and other manual therapies, my gratitude to my dear professional colleagues—Gillie Angoluan, Robert Morelli and Robert Taylor—who provided constructive advice about the direction for the book contents that would meet the needs of those groups.

Seventh, our designers. They created the visual concepts, including the shapes and colours and thus, the physical attraction and layout for communicating the information. So I can't thank Elina Mer enough for her patience and imagination in meeting my expectations for an effective book cover design. As well, I appreciate the advice of Joan Leacott who, in the interior book design department, helped me successfully manage the intricacies of word processing using Microsoft Word.

Last but not least, my greatest appreciation to my wife, Elaine for her diligent editing, and children, Keith and Karen, who have been totally supportive of this project and were so patient when I talked enthusiastically and endlessly about the need to educate the public about osteopathy. In fact, the unique design idea for the cover originated from a conversation with Karen.

INTRODUCTION

There's a sign in front of a chiropractor's office facing Highway 7, near Kipling Avenue in Vaughan, Ontario, that speeding motorists on their way to Brampton, a city north-west of Toronto, often miss. The glass-and-board sign, which is a stone's throw from my office, says in capital letters: "[Good] Health is a Natural State of Being."

If anyone takes those words to heart, it can mean that disease—along with the pain and other issues that often accompany it—is unnatural. Diseases are caused by the enemies inside the body. These no-good forces seem always ready to attack at any time and, according to osteopathy professionals, appear as disturbances within tissues and organs or misplaced body energies.

In osteopathy, the term "imbalances"—whether they are chemical, physical, emotional—is a catch-all phrase to describe those conditions.

Without taking care of these imbalances early on, one may get sick and experience accompanying pain and discomfort. Some people who say they are sick most of the time might, unfortunately, explain away their misfortune as the price they must pay for being on our planet.

When people with short- or long-term pain, whether mild or debilitating, are not getting relief from *allopathic medicine*—the conventional medicine administered by medical doctors—it may be time for them to consider the wide range of *natural medicine* options.

As an Ontario-based osteopathic manual practitioner (OMP)—one of two types of osteopathic practitioners, and a provider of natural medicine services—I believe osteopathy can help people, in most cases, obtain permanent relief from their "sick" situation and experience a better quality of life. The osteopathic way is holistic: it is founded on the proven idea that the body is self-healing. The human body is highly intelligent and resilient. It has the ever-present capacity to heal itself under the right conditions.

After osteopathic manual practitioners have listened to their patients' stories about their ailments, they use their finely tuned manual skills to "palpate" the body's internal and external systems to not only determine the root causes, but more importantly, to provide manual treatment and lifestyle advice in order to remove the imbalances and facilitate healing.

The other type of osteopathic practitioners in Canada—called DOs, or osteopathic physicians or doctors of osteopathic medicine—are also trained to use palpation and manipulation skills for diagnostic and treatment purposes.

However, because of their in-depth training in conventional medicine, they rarely use their osteopathic manual skills. More often than not, they favour conventional techniques using blood testing, X-rays and so forth, and for treatments, they rely almost entirely on prescribing drugs and performing surgery.

We, in the natural medicine professions—osteopaths, acupuncturists, chiropractors, naturopaths, traditional Chinese medicine practitioners, and dozens of others—are often asked: What is the role of medical doctors?

As osteopathic manual practitioners, we believe medical doctors are spot-on when it comes to diagnosing disease and treating patients based on signs and symptoms. But sometimes those signs and symptoms may be the body's reaction, or compensation, to make up for something else happening in another part of the body. So, when medicines are prescribed, they don't always solve the root cause of the problems. Since no health care provider of any kind has a monopoly on knowledge, osteopathic manual practitioners partner with medical doctors to ensure that patients obtain the best that all medical technologies can offer. This is called "integrative medicine."

We also partner with other natural health-care providers. This is called either "complementary and alternative medicine,"(CAM) or "alternate and complementary medicine"(ACM).

Chantal Roy, an Ottawa-based osteopathic manual practitioner understands the collaborative approach to helping her patients. She told the authors, "I think we have a good place among the others. I don't think we are the only professionals who can treat people."

Brad McCutcheon, an osteopathy professor at the Canadian College of Osteopathy, also emphasizes the value of collaboration in his practice: "We need to understand when osteopathy can apply to certain conditions and when it can't, and when to refer out and when not to."

Currently, in Canada, osteopathy is gaining popularity among medical and other health-care practitioners and the public.

Since the 1980s, osteopathic manual practitioners have successfully treated millions of Canadians for a wide variety of ailments. However, these osteopaths have yet to achieve regulatory status.

Doctors of osteopathic medicine have, by contrast, obtained limited recognition from medical regulatory bodies in several Canadian jurisdictions. Before they are issued medical licences to practise like regular medical doctors, however, they must satisfy other screening requirements.

Recently, word has it that Quebec is seriously considering a process that would likely lead towards regulation of osteopathic manual practitioners. It is appropriate to salute the Office des professions du Québec, the provincial government's health professions advisory agency, for its foresight. This initiative would likely help guarantee that Quebecers will have access to obtain a more ethical and safer osteopathic health-care system. When that happens, Quebec will be the first jurisdiction among the ten provinces and three territories to do so.

I hope, as a DOMP in Ontario, that in my lifetime, a health regulatory college, created under the *Regulated Health Professions Act* (1991), to govern manual practitioners, will be legislated into existence in my home province. In the meantime, the osteopathic movement in Ontario is conducting campaigns aimed at "educating" the politicians, health-care policy managers, and the general public about its standards of education, ethical code, and best practices to protect the public.

Atily Gunaratne

AMP, DPT, DOMP
Osteopathic Manual Practitioner

WHY THIS BOOK?

Thinking Hands was written to enlighten the general public about osteopathy and its benefits. It will also be of interest to osteopathic manual practitioners, osteopathic physicians and students, as it provides some back-stories about osteopathy's development in the provinces and territories in Canada. For graduating students, and future cohorts of practitioners, in particular, there are two reasons why this book is important.

First, knowledge of osteopathic events and people in the past is considered a core competency in the training benchmarks developed by the World Health Organization (WHO).

Second, to borrow the title of the once-popular 1973 movie starring Barbara Streisand and Robert Redford, *The Way We Were*, these four words provide an impetus for practitioners to spark further conversations about agreeing on the future direction for Canadian osteopathy.

Chapter 1 briefly explains the nature of manual osteopathy and its relationship to the dozens of other natural medicine systems and modalities. In chapters 2 through 14, the medical situations involving fourteen individual patients who had consultations about their ailments and subsequent osteopathic treatments from the author, an OMP based in Vaughan, Ontario, are described.

After each patient's case history, there is a short clinical commentary which includes the treatment plan that was developed for the patient as well as notes on the progress and/or outcome achieved.

The case histories range from a child with a lingering nightmare disorder to a boy who, for many years, couldn't eat pizza and other foods that tweens love having, to a woman who had an unenviable incontinence problem (all the food she ate—breakfast, lunch and dinner—would literally go right through her digestive tract within an hour or so), to the man who experienced double vision when he attended live theatre.

Like politics and other spheres of life, there are some controversies regarding osteopathy. The detractors claim osteopathy is not based on science. Some have even declared that manual osteopaths are into hocus-pocus remedies.

A good example of the misperceptions is this Internet-published evaluation of a single treatment administered to a patient in Mississauga in 2014. He wrote these unflattering remarks on a website and they are reproduced below in its entirety:

> I went to this 'doctor' (B.Sc., PT., DOMP, Doctorate in Osteopathic Manual Practice) with a chronic lower back pain. All he did was lay me down on a bed for an hour. He inspected somehow my body with his palms, and told me that this is something with my duodenum and my bile not functioning properly because I had too much wine during Christmas . . . which doesn't make sense no matter how tolerant I try to be. After that he tried to convince me that I feel better than when I came in, and then charged me $120. To me it looked like straight mumbo-jumbo this 'osteopathic manual practice'. Will never go to him again.[1]

While I felt a strong sense of empathy with this patient, given his longstanding medical issue, he and I, unfortunately, have had no continuing contact to discuss his concerns or review the results of the single treatment he received. Recovery from a chronic medical condition, after all, does usually require a reasonable time to take place.

A fairly well-known critic of alternate medical systems, therapies and techniques, is the main operator of the *Quackwatch* website (http://www.quackwatch.com/). Dr. Stephen Barrett, a retired psychiatrist, says he is concerned about health-related frauds, myths and fads, and since 1993 has launched a tirade against hair analysis, chiropractors, osteopaths and just about every other every health profession except psychiatry.

He has apparently failed to acknowledge the positive outcomes for millions of patients around the world who have benefited from alternate medical systems and therapies. Let it, therefore, be said that the patients are always and will be the final judges and juries.

Moreover, it must be remembered that the science of osteopathy has its own body of evidence-based knowledge dating back more than 150 years, and is part of our society's accepted medical knowledge system.

It is hoped that this "little book" will make a meaningful contribution to the storehouse of information on how osteopathy has helped with the health concerns of Canadians.

A.G.

TABLE OF CONTENTS

PART 1

OSTEOPATHY—A COMPLEMENTARY MEDICAL
SYSTEM

CHAPTER 1—OSTEOPATHS' HANDS 'PALPATING' PAIN AWAY

When you crave mussels and wish you were downing them in an "all-you-can-eat" establishment, downtown Halifax's Five Fishermen Restaurant's mussel bar could well be a good choice. The selection of sauces for its fresh water clams are as many and varied as the salad dressings.

When you are in pain, you could perhaps manage it through an "all-you-can-use" strategy by availing yourself of the multitude of naturally-based pain relief options available in Canada.

Pain relief agents of the holistic kind—and the alternate and complementary medicine practitioners who are skilled at prescribing the appropriate ones—are plentiful.

You can select from among several alternate medical systems such as Ayurveda, Chiropractic, Naturopathy and Osteopathy.

Or you can choose from various therapies and techniques such as body movement programs, creams, herbs and other botanicals, imagery, oils, over-the-counter drugs, sounds, prayer, and other spiritual activities. These are all touted as being able to reduce pain—ranging from acute pain due to nerve damage and tissue damage (such as muscle aches, tension, cramping, arthritis, and joint inflammation) to chronic pain due to the same causes but persist because of stress, fear, or anxiety.

And the professionals who calculate and calibrate how much and how many of these remedies patients should receive, run the gamut: from chiropractors, osteopathic manual practitioners, prayer-for-chronic pain facilitators, to "Trager Approach" experts, yoga gurus, and the dozens of other professionals who have expertise in providing pain relief.

Canadians have turned, at one time or another, to the following natural medical therapies—by no means, an exhaustive list—for non-emergency acute and chronic pain and illnesses.

Alternate medical systems which include: Ayurveda, Chiropractic, Homeopathy, Naturopathic medicine, Osteopathy, and Traditional

Chinese medicine.

Biologically-based therapies which include: Aromatherapy, Folk/Herbal remedies, Essential Oils therapy, High Dose/Mega Vitamins programs, Holistic (or Natural) nutrition, Special diets/Lifestyle diets.

Body-based therapies which include: Acupuncture; Body Work (such as Mitzvah Technique, Alexander Technique, and Feldenkrais Method), Colonic Irrigation, Dance and Movement therapy, Lymphatic therapy, Massage (such as government-regulated massage therapy, Swedish, Shiatsu), Reflexology, Energy therapies, Bach Flower remedies, Intuitive Arts, Magnet therapy, Meditation, Qigong, Reiki, Sound Energetics, Therapeutic Touch (such as the Trager Approach).

Mind-Body Techniques which include: Biofeedback, Emotional Healing, Hypnosis, and Imagery.

Osteopaths' Use of Palpation and Manual Manipulation

Chiropractic, physiotherapy, massage and osteopathy are bedfellows in two ways. They not only share a philosophy that recognizes the importance of the spine but also involve the practitioners' hands in diagnosing and treating patients.

While the public generally understands what massage therapists and physiotherapists do, the picture, for them, is not always clear about the roles of osteopathic practitioners and chiropractors. Often, the perception is that they are the same. In fact, each is a horse of another colour.

Chiropractors do "adjustments," says a team of British chiropractors on their website. These adjustments "are as specific as possible and aimed at restoring joint position and function. [But] osteopaths' typically take a broader approach and may treat a larger area."[2] Osteopaths use palpation (the process of using their hands to examine the body) as skillfully as medical doctors who place stethoscopes on patients to diagnose and determine the source of a medical problem.

But osteopaths' hands go beyond diagnosing; they treat the bodily systems to create a change in the patient's body structure and function, thus helping in the healing process.

Specifically, the osteopath's hands manipulate patients to:

- make sure that blood flow to tissues or organs become barrier-free, and
- boost the strength of the tissue or organ structure.

While doing these tissue manipulations, osteopaths are constantly bearing in mind that body parts are interdependent. So they treat the body as one unit.

Here's a glimpse of what happens when an osteopath is diagnosing and treating a patient:

Observing the patient from head to toe, even before using his/her hands, the osteopath can often determine what bodily systems are working below their optimum efficiency.

The osteopath may then place his/her hands gently on key areas of the body to gather information and correct any faulty structures using many techniques available in his/her repertoire. Sometimes, the osteopath may keep the hands in the same position on one spot for minutes at a time, before placing the hands on other areas of the body.

At this stage, the patient would not know whether the osteopath's hands are diagnosing or treating the body to reduce or eliminate the source of the ailment. Where the osteopath's hands are placed, how long they would remain on selected areas of the body, and how much pressure is applied by the hands (in osteopathy, pressure is minimal and some would say "always gentle") vary according to the osteopath's diagnosis and choice of treatment.

The various hand techniques used may be cranial, sacral and osteo-articular. Other types of techniques may include the use of muscle energy, visceral and myo-fascial release, and facilitated positional release.

Effective hand techniques trigger positive changes within the musculoskeletal, digestive, reproductive, cardio-vascular, respiratory and nervous systems of the patient. These changes affect not only the local area, but the body as a whole.

The goal of osteopathy's manual manipulations is to emphasize restoring the structural integrity of the body.

Worth Remembering

Osteopathy and other natural health-care systems and practices are effective complements to modern medicine. As Ontario osteopathy professor Brad McCutcheon once said—and his words are worth re-broadcasting—"We need to understand when osteopathy can apply to certain conditions and when it can't, when to refer out [to both medical doctors and other natural medicine practitioners] and when not to."

PART 2

ONTARIO CASE HISTORIES ILLUSTRATING OSTEOPATHIC MANUAL TREATMENTS

The following 13 chapters present case histories that provide an idea of the wide range of the work an osteopath does.

Each patient's case analysis has been described briefly. This is deliberate, as it is beyond the scope of this book to attempt detailed descriptions of how osteopaths diagnose and create a treatment plan.

It should be mentioned, however, that all the treatments prescribed were carried out following a detailed assessment of the whole patient, irrespective of the presenting symptoms and details of investigations.

The variety of cases illustrates how a global approach works in treating patients, *as opposed to direct treatment of symptoms*.

The treatment protocol described in each case history was designed according to the hierarchy of the lesion patterns. The frequency of treatments that was determined for each patient varied according to the acuteness of the problem.

The names that were used for the patients are fictitious in order to protect their identities but the cases are true stories as narrated by the patients.

CHAPTER 2—THE CASE OF HELENA DELL AND HER JAW

After my first treatment, I was still iffy about it. He [the osteopath] had these gentle hand movements and it felt like he wasn't doing anything. Actually over time, I saw and felt progress and how it helped me. It got to this point where it is better.

By the end of 2015, Helena Dell will have completed her third year as a full-time student in the University of Guelph-Humber degree program. She's looking forward with boundless enthusiasm to involving herself in behind-the-scenes work in the movies and television industries.

Two years earlier, however, thoughts about her post-graduation life would be few and far between. And that wasn't because she was in her frosh year. and had to adjust to the rigours of a college environment life.

The fact was that she had been feeling jaw pain from morning to night almost every day.

This discomfort wasn't anything new; she had been experiencing it since 2011 when she had completed the prescribed term for the metal braces she wore for three years to straighten her crooked teeth. With the orthodontic appliance out of her mouth, she was looking forward to smiling confidently again. She confessed she hadn't liked smiling naturally because she felt "self-conscious" of the silver braces on her front teeth.

So while the permanent removal of her braces marked the end of an aesthetics issue, it also marked the beginning of a medical problem.

Soon after, she remarked, "I started noticing my jaw clicking. I didn't think it was a big deal, and it would lock sometimes. Then at the beginning of 2013, it started locking and the jaw never was completely open again."

Before her lower jaw almost locked down totally, Helena recalled, "My mom referred me to a massage specialist she knew, but he was really aggressive. It hurt and it was painful. It was almost as if I was at the chiropractor's. My parents were really trying to get solutions for me. My dentist even suggested I might need to get braces again and NightGuard to fix it.

"My parents didn't know what to do," she said with a grim face in an interview, recounting her predicament. "My dad was concerned. He said to me, 'Do whatever is right and get whatever treatment you want!' and he would pay for it. He just wanted to get it fixed.

"It made my life difficult especially eating and talking. It's not noticeable to other people. But I could feel it in my mouth. I could talk, though. I was able to open my mouth halfway but it made eating difficult and that bothered me the most. I couldn't eat tough food like meat, and I couldn't eat pizza."

Her siblings couldn't help much. "My older brother was worried. My younger brother was five and he didn't understand what was happening," she said.

Turning to her aunt for advice, Helena got a referral to an osteopathic practitioner through her dentist. Describing her first visit to the osteopath, Helena said:

"He used a lot of medical language I didn't understand but he was trying to explain to me how connected the entire body is, so that it's not just my jaw that is the problem and that I need to fix it. It's like something I need to correct in my entire body. He gave me a lot of information and he seemed, out of all the other doctors and massage therapists I've seen, to be the one; he knew my case and knew what to do and knew what was wrong. I trusted him the most and that's why I continued to see him.

"In a lot of sessions, he was just quiet, his eyes closed, and he was making these tiny movements with his hands. But then at the end of it, I started feeling a big difference. Five treatments over four months. I haven't been back since. I don't feel I have anything to go back for," Helena declared.

The patient's name has been changed to protect her identity.

Commentary on Helena's Health Situation

Helena was referred to me by a dentist with whom I had previously discussed treatment options for temporomandibular (TMJ) problems.

Helena experienced locking of her mouth soon after the removal of her dental appliance. Another appliance was prescribed but the mouth started to get even stiffer and eating became a problem. Helena wore the night splint for one year without any relief.

When she arrived at the clinic I noted that her mouth opening was limited to about 10mm and it deviated to the left. Helena had to make a real effort to align the jaw. I explained to her that the left side of the jaw does not open fully and the right side compensates for it. There were also problems in the neck and the cranial bones.

In normal circumstances, the body naturally introduces compensatory mechanisms or adaptations. Through surgeries, injuries or dentistry we can lose our adaptations, however, and the body is unable to function freely.

Helena's left temporal bone was limited in mobility (cranial and facial bones do move as much as the rest of the body; it is, however, a subtle movement). Lack of mobility of this bone reduces the mobility of the ipsilataral temporomandibular joint, which in turn causes the contralateral TMJ to open more than it should. After Helena's left temporal bone was mobilized (spheno-petrous, petro-basilar and occipito-mastoid sutures and jugular foramen using functional techniques) along with other cranial, facial and cervical bones (zygoma, occiput, first cervical vertebra using facilitated positional release techniques and left TMJ again using functional techniques) the TMJ returned to normality.

Helena also had a mild scoliosis which we were able to correct. Her scoliosis was at the thoracolumbar junction with a compensatory curve in the cervicothoracic spine. This was a transient scoliosis due to connective tissue tightness in the duodenum area (part of the small intestine). Myofascial release techniques were administered to correct the scoliosis. Altogether, Helena had five treatment sessions.

As we know, the beginning of the digestive tract is the mouth and the other end is the anus. Any tightness along this tract (which is possible during formation of the organ) can show imperfections in the mouth due to uneven forces. Hence Helena may have had imperfect teeth. The scoliosis was to accommodate the length of the GI tract. The scoliosis transmitted forces to the opposite occipito-mastoid joint and reduced its mobility causing left temporal bone dysfunction.

CHAPTER 3—THE CASE OF JACK JACKSON AND HIS STOMACH

I was 9 years old. I visited my osteopathic guy for my gastroparesis which is a digestive problem. I had a one-hour appointment with the osteopathic doc once every two weeks. Basically he just touched my stomach area and in a couple of years it cleared up.

Preschoolers at age four talk a lot. The amount of their verbal expressions increases at that time of their lives. So when Jack Jackson was at that age, living in Hamilton, Ontario, with his mother and sister, he frequently used the words "I have to throw up!"

That was because he was suffering with gastroparesis, the medical condition when the stomach takes too long to empty the food inside it.

"It started when I was four when I was throwing up a lot. Pretty much everything," said Jack, now seventeen. "Eventually I started eating yogurt all the time. Yogurt didn't make me throw up. I also ate tons of peanut butter sandwiches and that didn't make me throw up. So I ate those two foods all the time as lunch and dinner for a very long time."

Jack recalled that in his preteen years in that then steel mill town, his teachers and peers had to cope with his numerous trips to the washroom. This went on for at least five years and his teachers and peers never got accustomed to the class interruptions.

"The teachers would actually get mad at me and shout at me for that. It wasn't even something I could control. And I was young. It was a bad experience".

Visiting a Pizza Pizza store or going to McDonald's was not particularly a bonding experience with his friends. "I'd tell them I don't eat pizza. And I don't like hamburgers," Jack would say to his friends all the time. "I think my friends believed me. They also probably thought I was a little weird because everyone likes pizza."

Jack also remembered vividly how a doctor used to give him some "awful" medicine to drink every day, and how it didn't help him feel better.

The doctor also told Jack he was suffering with a stomach condition for which "there was no cure" and that social life would suffer a great deal.

One day, when Jack was nine, a recommendation turned the tide of his life. Jack's mother, Lucille, heard about "some interesting work being done by an osteopath in Vaughan," said Jack. So she took Jack to consult the osteopath.

According to Jack, "I had a one-hour appointment with the osteopathic doc once every two weeks. Basically he just touched my stomach area and in a couple of years it cleared up."

Today, Jack declares about his digestive issue: "Right now, more than seven years later, no problem."

The patient's name has been changed to protect his identity.

Commentary on Jack's Health Situation

I had been seeing Jack's mother for her neck pain and headaches. During one of her sessions, she asked whether I could help her son who vomits almost after every meal. She explained that, at night, he had to sleep in an elevated position and that he was under the care of a gastroenterologist in Hamilton. I wanted to do an assessment first before I could say anything to her.

So Jack came with his mother one day to the office wearing a patch on his right eye. I was told this was designed to stimulate the left "lazy" eye. I was told he was taking domperidone to reduce reflux. On assessment I noticed he had limitation of his left temporomandibular joint along with the left temporal bone and left orbit. His left eye lid was drooping. This may indicate a dysfunction of nerves innervating the muscle cranial nerves III, IV, and VI. The joints in the left eye socket were restricting the nerves (superior orbital fissure). The left temporal bone's position was held in a closed way, compromising the space between the occipital and the temporal bones (jugular foramen). This is the space that permits exiting of the tenth cranial nerve, or vagus nerve, from the brain. The function of the digestive track depends on a proper nerve supply. A compromised nerve will negatively impact the function of the organs it innervates.

Jack's situation required long-term treatment from more than one health-care practitioner. He needed osteopathic treatments to correct the left temporal bone. The left jugular foramen was normalized with functional techniques to remove the restriction of the vagus nerve. Jack's sphenoid was treated to normalize the greater and lesser wing relationship. He required long-term manual treatments as he was growing and his tissues were changing. In addition, he required counselling because he had come to associate his mother's food with the need to vomit. He also required eye therapy to strengthen his eye muscles.

Jack's problems were successfully resolved following long-term treatments.

CHAPTER 4—THE CASE OF LEONID ANATOV AND HIS EYESIGHT

Russian doctors have told me this is rare and it does not give me any problems outside the theatre; it only happens after I go and see live theatre.

Leonid Anatov lives in Russia's second largest city and enjoys watching local movies. So when he flies into Ontario from Saint Petersburg occasionally to see his daughter and her family in Toronto, he sometimes accompanies them to see a Hollywood action film at a local Cineplex movie theatre.

But he reminds his family—although they know it—that he'd prefer not to go with them to the opera, theatre for kids and family, or musicals.

No, it's not that Leonid only watches movies and doesn't appreciate the fine arts which involve live performers, music and sets. Leonid has been suffering with "double vision" or diplopia, the medical term that refers to when a patient can't see a single, clear image of something.

But Leonid's diplopia is truly unique.

"Since I was a young boy I've been going to live theatre with my parents. The problem is that after seeing a live indoor performance I get 'double vision,'" said Leonid, a chemical engineer in his fifties.

"But I don't get double vision going to the movies, driving or being at home. I lecture in a university, and there is no problem there also. I play ping pong and there are no problems there either."

As a very analytical person, Leonid came to the conclusion only recently that traditional medicine can't help him; he now believes in the healing power of his body with intervention from osteopathic practitioners.

His Russian doctors hadn't been of much help. He added, "They see no problem with it if it only comes on with going to the theatre. They even said to me 'don't pay attention to it' and said 'you just need to get some more relaxation after seeing a show and then go home.'" Leonid noticed his vision wasn't right as a youngster attending live theatre in downtown

Saint Petersburg with his parents. He repeatedly told his parents about the problem. "But they didn't take me seriously. It was only when I turned forty, I began to look for solutions."

"After two sessions with Dr. Atily in 2011, this problem that I had for more than forty years, went away but only for half a year. It came back after I went to the dentist. There I had to open my mouth for a whole hour and I think that is why the double vision problem came back," said Leonid.

"So I went back to see Dr. Atily soon after. The treatment helped but it didn't go away totally like it did before. The double vision went away eighty per cent. So it's much , much better than before."

The patient's name has been changed to protect his identity.

Commentary on Leonid's Health Situation

Double vision occurs when both eyes cannot focus on an object.

This happens due to one or all of the III, IV AND VI cranial nerves having palsy (affected by paralysis). It can happen due to neoplasms (tumours), aneurysms or simply mechanical pressure on the nerves. These nerves enter the eye socket through an opening called the superior orbital fissure in the eye socket. It is comprised of lesser and greater wing of sphenoid (bones of the cranial base).

Since Leonid has had this problem for more than 40 years, it was safe to assume that there was no underlying medical problem. I examined his facial, cranial and cervical bones and re-established the relationship of the facial and cranial bones through cranial manipulative techniques which relieved his symptoms.

Once he returned to the dentist I assume, through the continuous opening of the mouth, the sphenoid bone resumed its lesion position or the malposition that it was used to (tissue memory).

Since this problem existed most of his life, I was of the opinion that when he was a child, he might have sustained an injury at the front of the head, or he sustained an injury during a forceps delivery at birth. For this reason it required follow-up treatments to re-educate the tissue. I advised him to seek follow-up treatments in his native country.

CHAPTER 5—THE CASE OF PRIYA HENDERSON AND HER IMMOBILITY

I couldn't even walk after the birth of my son. I hobbled around for many months and wasn't able to go back to work. I was unable to work or move around. I used a cane for walking.

Giving birth can be one of the happiest and most powerful events in the life of a woman. But for Priya Henderson, it triggered a chain of events that not only caused her a lot of physical pain but also temporary frustration about the ability of traditional health-care clinicians to diagnose and provide a medical solution.

"I couldn't even walk after the birth of my son. I hobbled around for many months and wasn't able to go back to work. I had to use a cane for walking," said Priya, a physiotherapist.

Her retired father, who travelled almost every day from Oakville to her small apartment in Mississauga to help, was a godsend. Her father's presence meant her husband was able to go to work regularly. Her inability to walk stumped every type of health-care practitioner she turned to. "The physiotherapist and chiropractor I had seen were unable to help. I also went to conventional doctors. They too couldn't figure it out," said Priya.

As a practising physiotherapist, she invoked her own professional storehouse of knowledge to pinpoint the source of the pain but the answer eluded her.

Her medical doctors gave her painkillers which she took only when she had to move around. "The pain only happens then, so I basically had to stay put most of the time."

In the months following the birth, Priya was on maternity leave from the clinic where she worked. Her daily routine after having the baby—going to the fridge, warming up milk at the stove and changing diapers and so on—was accompanied with pain, but, as a mother with unconditional love for her child, she coped with it.

For some time she wondered when the bouts of pain would end. When the baby was asleep, she naturally would reminisce about all the things she used to do with her husband and her friends.

Priya then turned to Dr. Atily whom she had met at a physiotherapists' seminar in Toronto years before.

"I'd have to say that during that year, Dr. Atily saved my life. In fact, I'd credit both Dr Atily and osteopathy for my recovery," Priya said.

As a professional health-care provider, Priya said she believes "that osteopathy is starting to become mainstream and as more and more people are living with chronic conditions, whatever that helps them, they will go for it.

"Each time I saw him and got treatment, things got a little better. After weekly treatments for about three months, I was myself again. And that's why I said it was pretty amazing."

The patient's name has been changed to protect her identity.

Commentary on Priya's Health Situation

I met Priya at a seminar I was presenting to the local physiotherapists' association. Priya came up to see me after the seminar to inquire more about osteopathy. Following that, she came to my office for some treatments.

Long after that, she contacted me after her first child was born. When she arrived at my office, she was at her wit's end with severe back pain and general body pain following the birth. She explained she had been seeing chiropractors and physiotherapists for the problem, but to no avail. She was unable to walk without a quad cane (a cane with four prongs) and had been spending most days in bed or lying down on a couch.

In my assessment, I noted that her pelvis was poorly aligned. Priya wore a belt that was given to her by the chiropractor to contain the sacrum. It gave her a sense of stability but did not allow pain relief.

She had dislocated a joint (symphysis pubis) in the front of her pelvis during labour but the joint did not return to its proper position following birth (normally the symphysis pubis will permit exit of the baby and return to its normal position after birth). There were visceral adhesions limiting the mobility of her pelvis. It was not possible to adjust the joint without preparing the muscles, ligaments and visceral contents. It required several visits to prepare and adjust the pelvis to facilitate complete relief.

Having done the needful, I reassured her that the second pregnancy would likely be all right and the risk of post-delivery pains would be low.

I followed her case until her next pregnancy and delivery. She did not experience further problems.

CHAPTER 6—THE CASE OF JENNY JONES AND HER DIGESTIVE AND OTHER PAINS

The first set of pains in my neck and shoulder started in Dominica where I lived as a teen. While there I also had stomach pain. They had diagnosed me with peptic ulcer. The doctors there took me off fried foods to deal with it. When I came to Canada, I didn't follow the strict diet that I used to follow when I was a teen. My stomach problems continued.

Do you ever remember, by chance, seeing a woman in Toronto, years ago, holding up her head with her hands while walking along the street?

If you did, it could have been Jenny Jones. No, it wasn't because she was trying out moves as a potential busker. She literally had to do what she did; she couldn't do otherwise unless she wanted to feel the pangs of pains that have dogged her for years.

Jenny's health issues started way back in Dominica when she was a teen. When she first came to Canada in her twenties she gave up on her strict diet that controlled her ulcer pains.

When she started working in her early thirties, things changed. "I started getting pains in my neck, shoulder, and even down my spine, and they started getting worse. You wouldn't believe this but I used to hold up my head while walking. Driving my car was really, really hard," Jenny recalled. Enjoying her life after a work day was often denied her.

The idea of working out in a gym was unthinkable. She was even afraid to walk or run because of the pain.

What was worse was the traditional medical folks were not able to provide a solution.

"All this time I had been seeing MDs and medical specialists who gave me painkillers and ulcer pills and they all had different ideas about what could be causing my pains," Jenny explained. "I also saw chiropractors, masseurs and physiotherapists and it wasn't helping with lessening the pains. I saw these health care professionals almost every week for four years."

The road to resolving this longstanding issue was found at her job at a Toronto university where she also studied human resources management.

Part of the story she related to us goes like this:

"One time, a professor, who passes by my desk once a week, says to me, 'You always seem to be in so much pain.' So I explained to her what had been happening to me for years. She then said to me, 'I have someone I want you to meet'. The female professor gave me contact information so I could meet with a west-end Toronto osteopath who had been working together with her surgeon-husband.

"After my third treatment session with him, I started getting some relief. Right away, I felt different with his treatment approach. Because I lived out of town, he referred me to Vaughan, Ontario – based Atily Gunaratne whom I saw in January 2011 for the first time and that was when my real journey with osteopathy began."

Today Jenny feels like she's a new person. "I've lost a lot of weight. I'm now able to drive without discomfort and to drop my daughter off for school, get to her basketball practice, and visit her friends' houses.

"Meeting Dr. Atily was the best thing that ever happened to me," Jenny said from her home in Vaughan. "Today, I feel just great. Never felt better. I've been seeing him regularly for two years now—sometimes weekly, sometimes every three weeks. The amazing thing about it was Dr. Atily's ability to make—and help me understand—the connection between my stomach and the pains I had been having in the rest of my body."

The patient's name has been changed to protect her identity.

Commentary on Jenny's Health Situation

When Jenny came to see me she was in severe pain in the neck/shoulder area. She told me she had only obtained temporary relief from various treatment modalities in the past. She also knew that her health was failing due to her stressful job and her household chores.

On examination, I noted that her body was swollen. From my assessment, I determined that Jenny was suffering from a metabolic as well as a right-sided temporomandibular dysfunction. She had some teeth missing due to extractions in early life. As well, she was dealing with food intolerances which helped cause her metabolic dysfunction. That part was easy to correct as Jenny was so eager to get better. She changed her diet, on my advice, and started to lose weight.

The neck problem was related to a petro-basilar joint (a dense bony joint at the base of the skull) dysfunction most probably from a tooth extraction that was performed years ago. It took some time to prepare the tissue around the neck and head before correcting the dysfunction. Cranial manipulation techniques were used.

Jenny was pain-free before she decided to have braces put on to correct the gaps left following the extractions. She complained about headaches and left-sided neck pains as well as discomfort on the left side of her body each time the braces had to be adjusted. I continued to monitor her periodically due to the fact that she had to wear the corrective appliance in the mouth for some time.

Jenny had also been involved in a motor vehicle accident during this period which complicated matters. She was experiencing more neck pains and headaches which were alleviated in additional treatment sessions.

CHAPTER 7—THE CASE OF MARY HARRINGTON AND HER TMJ

He was right. He was spot on. I did have an accident as a child. I had had trauma to my head and it affected me all my life with headaches.

Toronto salesperson Mary Harrington has often heard people say, 'Expect the unexpected!' and 'Didn't see that coming!' It isn't foreign to her. In fact, sometimes at her job, she finds her sales are sometimes much, much higher than she expected.

She's since discovered that anticipating and preparing for what she didn't think can happen are important.

In 2005, she was suffering with many ailments and decided to seek some help. She knew of a osteopathic practitioner that had successfully treated her husband so she decided to make an appointment and have some treatments.

Atily Gunaratne had hardly begun his assessment when he said to her, "You must have a lot of headaches—migraine headaches, right?"

According to Mary, Gunaratne told her that "just by the way I moved my jaw and the overall configuration of my face, he could tell I had probably been experiencing ongoing headache issues, that I possibly had a temporomandibular dysfunction.

"He was right. He was spot on. I did have an accident as a child. I had had trauma to my head and it affected me all my life with headaches."

She received treatments over a period of a few months and although she still gets tension headaches at times, her migraines have disappeared. "The treatments made a world of difference," said Mary.

"He recommended me to see a naturopath for my intestinal problems and it really helped me that he just focused on the fascial-skeletal work that he did," she explained. "I also had a problem with one hip, and he aligned it with the other so my body could become more symmetrical," Mary added. "My hip had not been a big deal really and did occasionally ache from time to time. But it was great that I got another benefit from getting osteopathic treatment."

"One of the good things about the medical people in osteopathy and naturopathy is that they help keep you healthier because they are proactive rather than others who are more reactive," Mary said.

"A few years ago in 2009, I developed some issues with my jaw and instead of going to see Atily, I went to see someone in mainstream medicine. That someone prescribed me some serious medication, like injecting me with some steroids. I didn't want that at all. So I contacted Dr. Atily again and got a few treatments. That helped a great deal," she added.

The patient's name has been changed to protect her identity.

Commentary on Mary's Health Situation

Mary came to the clinic in 2005 with a host of complaints. Among them were constipation during most of her life, temporomandibular joint (TMJ) pain for six years, headaches prior to using corrective dental bracing for three years, and a night splint. Her previous history included a head injury with a concussion at the age of 6 or 7.

Her cranial injury was the primary course of her headaches and TMJ pain. The appliances to correct the teeth had made the dysfunctional cranial bone problem worse.

Corrective techniques were applied to the head and neck (cranial-osteopathy). Because the cranial problem has been there since childhood, it required a series of treatments to realign the whole cranial and facial structure. Once a physiologically incorrect position is maintained due to trauma, the rest of the body adapts to maintain its physiology. Though this may not be the best position for the mechanical structure, it is necessary to maintain the homeostasis.

The mechanical structure of the body changes over time. After treatments, it starts to change slowly and regains normal positions. These changes are slower in older adults as opposed to children and young adults due to the growth factor. Mary was treated with muscle energy, osteo-articular, fascial and visceral techniques. I referred her to a naturopath to resolve her constipation.

She told me later that the osteopathy treatments and the consultations with the other therapist alleviated all her medical issues. When Mary returned to the clinic in 2009, she was suffering with neck pain associated with muscles of the neck and upper ribcage. The position of the neck was causing her TMJ pain. Mary was administered with osteopathic adjustments to her thorax, neck and clavicles to rebalance her. This time Mary required shorter treatment length as her body had regained a closer to normal physiological state of its skeletal structure.

Chapter 8—The Case of Kathy Wynn and Her Facial and Neck Pains

I had CT scans done on my brain to see whether I had an aneurysm or something. So in the first three months, nobody was able to figure out what was causing the pain

Life throws a curve ball at people. When that ball is in the direction of their personal health, they turn to health care professionals for a diagnosis and the start of a treatment plan to put them back on the road to wellness.

But sometimes many of those health-care folks are unable to figure out what's wrong.

Accountant Kathy Wynn found this out only too well in the months leading up to the autumn of 2011.

"In October of 2011, I had gotten some teeth taken out and later had Invisalign trays put in by my dentist to straighten my other teeth," said Kathy. "But I started having a lot of pain in my neck, arms, feet and head. For me, at that time, I couldn't believe my braces could cause that much pain. I couldn't touch my scalp and couldn't comb my hair. My face hurt too. I went to see a few doctors and they told me it was just 'stress.' Despite what they said, I felt there was something physically wrong with me. I had just changed jobs at the time it happened, so I went along believing it was stress," Kathy explained.

"So in the first three months, nobody was able to figure out what was causing the pain," Kathy recalled.

"I don't think anybody, like my employer, knew what was happening. Everybody, including my friends, was trying to figure out what was going on. I'd come home from work and just go to bed. I eventually stopped working and went on disability for a while. I couldn't go to work. All I could do was to stay in bed and take painkillers. I took a lot of painkillers. On a day-to-day basis I'd take things like Flexeril and Naproxen. About ten kinds of painkillers actually," she said.

"My massage therapist told me it could be my braces; my orthodontist said the cause wasn't because of the braces. Of course, I went to various MDs and so I was going back and forth," Kathy said with a frustrated voice.

"I told them how I was feeling, but nobody could give me a proper answer," said Kathy. "I knew something was seriously wrong with me. My alternative practitioners said I had TMJ. I had a splint put in my mouth to get a better balance—they thought I dislocated something in my mouth."

Close to Christmas Day in 2011, things became unbearable for her.

Kathy described this high point of her troubles this way: "It got really bad. I couldn't even feed myself and or could hardly open my mouth to eat Jello. I also lost a lot of weight. I'd go for days without eating. I couldn't eat food, I couldn't do anything. I was almost paralyzed.

"My parents were really concerned. They saw a complete change in my lifestyle," Kathy explained. "We had CT scans done on my brain to see whether I had an aneurysm or something."

But things turned around in the summer of 2012 when she visited an osteopathic manual practitioner in Vaughan, Ontario.

After five months of osteopathic treatment, Kathy reported that her facial pain, headaches and neck pain decreased. "I still now experience pain some days but it is not half as bad as before," she said.

The patient's name has been changed to protect her identity.

Commentary on Kathy's Health Situation

Kathy encountered an unfortunate situation in which a well-intended procedure by a health-care practitioner had major life-changing implications for her. She was told that the pains she was experiencing were "imaginary" and was given heavy doses of medication as well as being referred to a psychiatrist.

Her issue was, in fact, a dislocation of a small bone (the palatine) in the roof of the mouth. This might have happened during an extraction procedure for a tooth.

This particular bone, in its dislocated state, caused increased tension in the face, neck and the whole body. When the neck is not in the correct position, the rest of the body adjusts to maintain horizontal graze. Thus, the connective tissue throughout the body suffers to maintain the position thereby causing pain. So whenever Kathy turned her neck to one side, it would cause pain at the side of her neck and arm.

It took a few sessions of cranial and facial bone manipulations (cranial osteopathy and fascial release functional techniques were used in this case) to alleviate the fascial tensions throughout the body which had been there for months. Once all corrections were made by applying osteopathic manipulative techniques to the fascial chains, the palatine repositioned to its place of rest and the remainder of the body returned to its normal functioning.

CHAPTER 9—THE CASE OF MARISSA LANG AND HER LOWER BACK

Every medical doctor in Quebec I've ever seen has said to me more or less: 'Why don't you try these pills [pain killers].' I didn't think anything or anyone could help me.

The trauma people experience during and after a terrifying event often leads to a mental health condition called PTSD (post-traumatic stress disorder).

When communications consultant Marissa Lang moved to Toronto from Montreal, it was a great new life for her. But the effects of the accidents she had had as a child and at university remained with her after she crossed the Quebec-Ontario border.

Long after ditching her school bag, she felt her back was not right. "I couldn't stand for very long," she said. "I remember once when I was in a shopping mall and in a store I had to prop myself up against a clothing rack.

"You see, it was that bad!" she recalled.

"Every medical doctor in Quebec I've ever seen has said to me more or less: 'Why don't you try these pills [painkillers]' I didn't think anything or anyone could help me." Marissa said.

Recounting the history of her back, Marissa explained, "I had fallen down when I was at university and hurt my lower back. It really hurt. I was much younger then—in my twenties—and recuperated fairly quickly not thinking that down the line it might affect me later. "Even in high school, my back went out a few times. I remember one time when I reached under the bed, my back would hurt. But I still played in the badminton team, and took jazz and ballet."

Shortly before she moved to Toronto in 2002, her family doctor who was open to the idea of alternative medicine suggested she see an osteopath. At that time, she didn`t know fully what an osteopath did.

"So I saw one briefly, and when I got to Toronto, I went on the

Internet," Marissa remembered. "When I first started seeing Dr. Atily in Toronto, he told me my back had been sore and crooked because my kidney was pulling at it," she said.

"My back today is very good. Whenever I travel to Montreal and back and each trip takes five hours or so, my back doesn't bother me. Atily, the osteo guy, has really helped me straighten my back," said Marissa.

"What I also learned from him was how all the parts of the body interconnect. People may think the body works only mechanically but it also depends on things like what you eat. I've learned a lot about how the body works. I still see him every month. Initially, I was seeing him once a week for treatment."

In an interview, Marissa said: "Today, when I think back about the condition of my back more than a decade ago, I say to myself I was too young to have a back issue like that and to have experienced so much pain."

The patient's name has been changed to protect her identity.

Commentary on Marissa's Health Situation

Marissa was in agony at the time she consulted me for her severe back pain. She had already seen one osteopath in Toronto.

On examination, I noted Marissa had difficulty even just walking into my office and trying to stand upright. She was bent to the left side. There were tissue contractures on the left side and she had been gaining weight due to lack of exercise. Deep tissue under the ribcage was contracted.

It took many sessions to correct all underlying tissue contractures using osteopathic manipulative techniques. Once I manipulated all connective tissues that were contracted, they returned to their appropriate length allowing her to regain her natural mobility.

This required manipulation of all visceral connective tissues (using functional techniques) as well as the skeletal tissues (using facilitated positional release techniques).

I monitored her for months due to her other issues such as weight gain. I was able to use the services of an herbalist to reduce her weight and even her blood pressure came down to normal limits for her age.

Even after completing her treatment sessions, Marissa often consulted with me prior to her Toronto/Montreal trips to ask whether she could travel such a long distance.

Chapter 10—The Case of Palma Carboni and Her Neck

The doctor mentioned surgery. Right away I said to him "No, you're not doing surgery unless it's a life or death situation". I knew he didn't like what I said. So he changed his tone and said: "You know what. You're not in desperate need. You just have to exercise and you'll be fine."

On July 6, 2007, Palma Carboni was in a locked acrobatic position, assisting her employer, a dentist, while the patient, with his mouth wide open and his eyes closed, sat comfortably on the chair. She'd done this hundreds of times. That physical position would, as it turned out, mark a major juncture in her life.

By mid-morning, she felt something shift diagonally in her neck and then pain. "I knew it was not a kink. I got up from the chair I was sitting on, and the dentist asked me what was wrong. 'Something just happened,' I said to him. I thought maybe I was stressed out because at the time I was working long hours," said Palma. The pain didn't go away.

"On the following day, I felt I probably just needed to get some exercise. At the time I didn't think it was anything serious. So I went to my regular weekly aerobics class. But I couldn't do it. There was pain. I went to work the following Monday anyway, but didn't accomplish much. I felt limited in turning my neck. By Wednesday, six days later, I was seized up and I had tingling and numbness in my hands. I felt as if my shoulders were cemented to my ears; I couldn't turn at all," Palma said.

She described how the condition became protracted: "As the days went on, and the weekends came, it became worse and worse. As the pain increased, I found myself with even more limited mobility. Every time I met people they'd ask me 'what kind of accident were you in?' People couldn't understand what really happened to me. My parents were really concerned."

Palma also described the following weeks.

"I went to my massage therapist and she said there was something really wrong. She couldn't move anything. She said to me, 'You know what? You should get some acupuncture to move something.' The next day, I saw my naturopath who does acupuncture. The naturopath-acupuncturist told me later it took her a long time to put the needles in because I was so seized up. 'You're so seized up, I think you should go and see your chiropractor.'

"A week went by and I saw the chiropractor. I also went to the walk-in clinic so I could get a CAT scan. When the doctor got the test results, he told me: 'If you get worse or you can't breathe, you'd better go to a hospital emergency right away.'

"At that stage, when I touched my neck, I couldn't feel anything there. My doctor started telling me things like, 'if this happens or that happens, if you lose control of your bladder, etc.

"The doctor also talked about the possibility that I was suffering from cervical spondylolisthesis which is a problem with the upper spine. I was getting really scared, not knowing what's really going on. I looked at him and told him: 'Tell me what I need to do to get better! I am not going down that road!' At that time he wanted me to go and see a neurosurgeon. He mentioned surgery. Right away I said to him 'No, you're not doing surgery [on me] unless it's a life or death situation!' I knew he didn't like what I said. So he changed his tone and said: 'You know what? You're not in desperate need. You just have to exercise and you'll be fine.'

"In the meantime, no medications were working. Tylenol Two and Three, and even the pain killers my employer, the dentist, gave me didn't help. All these narcotics made me drowsy but I couldn't sleep. I also tried ice and the hot water bottle," said Palma recalling those months of pain.

One day, her massage therapist who had started her first year in osteopathic studies, suggested she try osteopathy. "I didn't know what osteopathy was—never heard of it!" Palma said.

After four years of treatment with osteopath Atily Gunaratne, Palma said she felt "so much better than when I first walked in the front door of his office. How I feel now is not a matter of a percentage but a matter of what I can do like turning my head. And when I walk I am much straighter than before.

"I would say if it weren't for him I would be in really bad shape. The label [accident victim] people gave me didn't mean anything to me. I just wanted to get relief. Now I'm happy just to be able to do half of the things I used to do. I used to go out to the gym a lot. Now it's just a simple little thing like I go to the pool to do some exercises [after treatment].

"My strength is increasing. You go on for so long in pain, and today, you can now see the more chummy side of me and I've come a long way since then," said Palma.

The patient's name has been changed to protect her identity.

Commentary on Palma's Health Situation

This was a challenging case of convincing someone that her neck pain was not just a neck pain but one that is connected to many parts of the body that were not functioning properly.

When I saw Palma for the first time, she looked like a tin soldier.

First, I was told by the receptionist she did not—and could not—sit on the waiting room chair. I knew then I was in for a challenge of my life. Thanks to my long-term experience, I requested her neck imaging results before I even touched it. Once I looked at the imaging, I told her that I could not treat her neck without treating the rest of the body. Luckily, Palma had no paralysis of muscles. Frankly, I was scared to touch her neck.

By the time she had come to me, she had had two years of therapy from a naturopath, a massage therapist, a chiropractor and a physiotherapist. She had also taken a lot of pain medications. I knew it was going to take a long time for her to reach a proper functional level. If I had videotaped her, we could today see the progress.

Examining her, I found she was very poorly nourished. Her digestive tract was dysfunctional. Her metabolic dysfunctions caused toxicity and adhesions throughout her body. The quality of tissue was very poor. She suffered from haemorrhoids and was unable to sit.

We discussed various treatment options, the first being a change in her diet to normalize her metabolic dysfunctions. Then I worked with the pelvis, sacrum and progressed by treating the spine and the rib cage. To achieve full function visceral manipulations were done to all visceral connective tissue.

To document Palma's whole treatment protocol will require a whole book, literally. Here I've documented only a small fraction of the treatments I administered.

CHAPTER 11—THE CASE OF LUCILLE CAPELLO AND HER HEADACHES

I was willing to give anything a try to see if it felt right.

Like the lower section of a river, the path that some follow to end up at the osteopath's door is often a meandering one.

Although an experienced children's book writer, Lucille Capello had never heard of osteopaths or osteopathy. It wasn't long after her dental braces and her temporomandibular joint (TMJ) dysfunction gave her days and nights of headaches, that she stumbled upon information about osteopathy.

This was the turning point for the mother of two. Talking with a friend who was a patient of a Vaughan osteopathic practitioner, she learned about "the wonderful things an osteopath can do to adjust a person's bodily structure."

She acted quickly on the information and is today headache-free and glad "I was willing to give anything a try to see if it felt right."

Lucille's tale of pain started when she saw an orthodontist to get braces.

"I went to the orthodontist because my teeth were misaligned. I didn't know my upper and lower teeth were rubbing at each other and it was getting worse," said Lucille. "I was also concerned about how my teeth looked."

"The dentist attempted to realign things with the braces and it worked for a little while but it all went bad," she recalled. "Sure, the teeth got straightened out with the braces and wires and once the braces were taken off, the teeth went back to their original position."

The patient's name has been changed to protect her identity.

Commentary on Lucille's Health Situation

Lucille is a friend of one of my clients. Lucille had heard from her that she could obtain relief from her neck pains and headaches.

Lucille's complaints were neck pain on the left side, headaches and temporomandibular pain which started following her cosmetic dentistry. Her past history also included being involved in four motor vehicle traffic accidents, a tonsillectomy and a broken toe. She had a mild thoracic scoliosis convex to the right side. There were corresponding curves in the cervical and lumbar spine.

Lucille had also suffered whiplash injuries during the traffic accidents, and these injuries had never been treated properly. The dental appliances probably made her existing problems worse. Aligning the teeth by bracing meant imposing a fixed point. This caused the body's natural compensations to be restricted. She was otherwise healthy.

The main objective in Lucille's treatment plan was to correct muscle imbalances. I applied osteopathic manipulative techniques to the affected connective tissues, including the cranium. This involved several treatment sessions. Lucille was happy she persisted with her visits as, with the passage of time, the cranial dysfunction that had been causing the headaches and neck pains cleared up.

CHAPTER 12—THE CASE OF SHEILA ABELLI AND HER ENCOUNTER WITH INCONTINENCE

I had to go to the bathroom about 10 to 15 times a day.

As a young woman in her early twenties, Sheila experienced the discomforts of IBS (irritable bowel syndrome) a common functional gastrointestinal (GI) disorder. With the help of natural health therapists like homeopaths, Sheila, an analyst at a Greater Toronto Area ceramic arts company, overcame the aches and discomforts of this affliction that affects about five million Canadians today.

Yet the worst was yet to come.

Fewer than seven years later, at the age of thirty with a husband and two kids, Sheila experienced another GI problem, perhaps the worst of about sixteen other common gastrointestinal disorders—fecal incontinence (FI).

Sheila described what happened to her: "If I ate anything, it would go right through me.

"After my second pregnancy with my son, I had fecal incontinence that I could not get rid of. I tried many different things that helped me diet-wise, health-wise, but I couldn't get to a point where it could stop happening," said Sheila.

But it did stop. But only after getting osteopathic treatment that capped eighteen months of visits to medical doctors including a GI specialist, a functional medicine practitioner, (a medical doctor who has a medical practice that considers treatments based on analysing the environment and how this may affect the body), a homeopath, and a nutritionist.

Looking back today, Sheila recalls, "It was horrible; I had a really rough time."

Her FI began about eight weeks after the birth of her second child and coincided with her having to return to work after maternity leave. "I went back to work with this issue," she said. "It's another issue when you have the issue around people. That was hard for me because you're going back to work after your leave and you have these problems."

"I had to go to the bathroom about ten to fifteen times a day," Sheila said. "When I went back to work, I was still seeing the GI doctor but he wasn't able to help me."

Then, on a subsequent visit to her functional medicine practitioner, things turned around. According to Sheila, the doctor said to her: "Despite all the tests I've given you for GI distress because your symptoms are GI related , nothing has showed up. So I think what's happening to you is more like an anatomy and physiology thing within your body that happened during your pregnancy. You need to be realigned and readjusted inside yourself."

The doctor knew of osteopathic practitioner Gunaratne, and he recommended that she see him, and off Sheila went to his office.

"After four treatments with osteopathy I felt a tremendous difference in my whole life," Sheila declared. "Now I am feeling so much better." But she admits a mild form of FI could come back once every six months "if I ate something I shouldn't be eating."

The patient's name has been changed to protect her identity.

Commentary on Sheila's Health Situation

Sheila was initially embarrassed to tell me the story of her fecal incontinence. Ever since she had her second child, she had no control over her bowel motions.

Sheila had seen every kind of practitioner to find relief. She had received rectal stimulation at the hospital in the hope of strengthening the sphincters, and also done Kegel exercises religiously as she was instructed to.

There was no improvement of her condition with those efforts. Finally, she visited a functional medicine specialist who knows me. This is how Sheila ended up in my office.

Sheila had suffered many years with IBS, and she had taken every precaution to avoid foods that would adversely affect her. On examination, I discovered her sphincter issue was related to the nerve input to the sphincter. The anal sphincter was not regulated as this is not a voluntary muscle. It is an involuntary autonomic function. I was able to mobilize the adhesions in the inferior mesenteric ganglion, the area that was causing the nerves to be compromised. In addition, the pelvic floor was treated to free the pudendal nerve. These adhesions were formed due to prolonged inflammation of her bowel due to IBS.

Prior to the birth of her child, Sheila's body managed to compensate well. But the body de-compensated, following her pregnancy, causing the nerve to be compromised. Once I removed the adhesions with osteopathic manipulations, her body was able to return to its normal physiological state.

CHAPTER 13—THE CASE OF JILL CARSON AND HER TROUBLE SUSTAINING A NORMAL PREGNANCY

I had to find out alternative ways to address my fertility issues.

Ask thirty-five-year-old Jill Carson what she remembers about the details she was told while consulting with health care professionals of all kinds during her four-year wait to have a normal pregnancy. Although a community college instructor with an excellent memory of the social sciences, she might say she doesn`t recall a lot but quickly reveals what she clearly remembers: the disheartenment she felt when her OB/GYN (obstetrician-gynaecologist) told her there was no reason why she couldn't become pregnant even though, she says, "I had a good egg reserve and my husband sperm count was above average for his age."

The back-story to Jill's normal pregnancy in 2014 is that she was indeed pregnant once before—in the middle of the summer of 2010. But it wasn't one of the good types; it was an ectopic one (that meant the fertilized egg attached to her fallopian tubes instead of her uterus).

"An ectopic pregnancy is deadly for the mother . . . I could have died," said Jill, explaining that she went as soon as possible to get a D and C (dilation and curettage – a surgical procedure used to remove uterine tissue after termination of a pregnancy).

It became evident that she was going to have a problem conceiving. So the next step for Jill and her husband was to try IVF (in vitro fertilization) therapy with a reproductive endocrinologist, a medical doctor who specializes in fertility issues. But her investment of $20,000 for a six-week cycle of IVF still killed her dream of having a family. It didn't work.

Jill and her husband's determination to get to the bottom of the issue saw them travelling regularly from their Oshawa home to various points around the Greater Toronto Area in search of solutions.

So over the next eight months, she—with her supportive husband accompanying her—began a journey of learning more about the "mind-body" connection. First, they engaged two naturopathic doctors in Oakville who put her on a special diet (gluten-free, non-GMO), performed rounds of acupuncture treatments and helped her with exercises to "balance the chi" (an Eastern healing practice that apparently heals the electromagnetic field generated by the body).

These visits also involved a cleansing. "I felt I needed to cleanse myself of the hormones" which she received through the conventional medical system. After a lot of reading, their decision to follow a holistic route was simple: "We decide we should step away from Western medicine." said Jill. "I had to find out alternative ways to address my fertility issues."

However, those encounters which lasted about eight months did not bring her closer to realizing her goal.

One day, a work colleague who had also experienced difficulty maintaining a pregnancy, including a miscarriage, suggested to Jill that she visit an osteopathic practitioner in Vaughan.

Following several osteopathic manual treatments in 2014, Jill was able to get pregnant. "I feel blessed and grateful to have been put in Dr. Atily's path," she said. She was told her baby would be expected in the spring of 2015. Happily, Jill's child arrived in the world in March 2015.

The patient's name has been changed to protect her identity.

Commentary on Jill's Health Situation

It was one of my most fulfilling experiences as an osteopath—analyzing the problem that Jill had which prevented her from maintaining a pregnancy.

In my initial assessment, I noted mainly that there were issues with her abdominal area, such as poor vitality of tissues. I could not find any major hormonal dysfunctions.

I asked her about any past head traumas. Jill could not recall any but she complained of headaches in the right eye area. When I further evaluated her head, I did notice a head trauma that had occurred sometime before.

Probing her memory, Jill recalled being in an accident in Mexico when she hit her head against the roof of a truck. That injury left her with a dysfunctional cranial suture called the parietal notch. This dysfunction caused her left temporal bone to be restricted in its motion and increased tension in the membranes which caused her pituitary gland to be compromised. In turn, this would affect her thyroid as well as other hormonal organs.

Once I treated the cranial lesion, the body returned to its homeostatic state.

This has been my experience with many of my clients who had fertility issues. While they are otherwise normal in their anatomy and physiology, they have a history of cranial injury.

Jill went through a normal pregnancy following the treatment and delivered a healthy baby nine months later at the exact due date.

I should mention that two days prior to her due date, Jill arrived at the office in a panicked state, saying that her baby has not dropped and they were planning a C-section. The C-section did not take place and I believe I assisted her in having a normal vaginal birth with the use of osteopathic manipulative techniques.

CHAPTER 14—THE CASE OF ANNA'S DAUGHTER, INGE, AND HER 'NIGHT TERRORS'

Often these situations would actually scare my husband and me.

Six-year-old Inge's doctor was right about one thing.

When young children, like Inge, experience Pavor Nocturnus, a sleeping disorder, also called night or sleep terror, they would probably grow out of it usually between ten and nineteen years of age, said the paediatrician, bluntly laying it out for Anna Cosenza, Inge's mother.

As her motherly instinct took hold, Anna was certainly not willing to have her perennially "bad skinned" second daughter with "an often off-temperament and behaviour" wait possibly four to thirteen years for nature to take its natural course. The magnitude of Inge's challenge and the specialist doctor's prediction were such that few—if any—mothers with the patience of Job in enduring suffering, would accept it comfortably.

Since age two-and-a half, the young Cosenza had hardly "slept well, she has had nightmares all the time," said Anna. "Inge would scream and yell for hours and hours. Sometimes, she would be screaming and we couldn`t get her to calm down. And these nightmares went on every week for four years."

Describing what happened when she and her husband, Tony, went into the room that Inge shared with her slightly older sister, Matilda, Anna said they would take her out of the room so the older one could get some sleep.

"Sometimes Inge would be asleep when she stopped yelling, sometimes she'd be awake with a blank look on her face, staring at the window and saying, 'I can't change the channel on the TV—why won't the station change,'" Anna recalled. Often these situations would actually scare her and her husband.

But early 2014, a change—of a different kind—took place.

Within a few days after the first osteopathic manual treatment at the

Osteopathic Health Centre in Vaughan, "Inge's screaming stopped a week after her first session with the osteopath," Anna claimed.

"She no longer has night terrors. If she has a nightmare it would be now once in a blue moon. When that happens she would wake up and be able to talk to me and tell me what's wrong—which wasn't the case before."

In 2014, Inge started grade one and according to her teacher, "she's a smart student and she's doing well," said Anna.

Young Inge continues to visit her osteopathic practitioner but not as frequently.

The patient's name has been changed to protect her identity.

Commentary on Inge's Health Situation

This is a very interesting case where this patient's primary complaint was not initially night terrors.

Inge was referred to me by a dentist to correct her posture. Inge had slight scoliosis and her feet were flat. It was, during my assessment, when I inquired about her birth history that her mother told me about the ongoing problem of night terrors.

On my examination, I also observed an indentation on her head which related to a forceps-assisted delivery. In my experience, those individuals who have had such a delivery or other induced delivery tend to suffer from headaches as they age. In the case of a forceps-assisted one, the pressure from the forceps would likely cause cartilaginous bones to sustain a strain pattern and thus reduce the fine mobility of the cranial bones. Further it causes the membranes inside to become imbalanced. This can, therefore, transfer throughout the cranium and spine to cause a scoliosis.

After treating her birth injury through cranial manipulative techniques, there were some remarkable results. Inge's night terrors disappeared, her appetite improved, her posture and scoliosis were corrected and her leg pains resolved.

PART 3

CANADIAN OSTEOPATHY HISTORY
FROM THE 1890S

CHAPTER 15—'THINKING HANDS' IN CANADA THROUGH THE DECADES

During the late 1890s and early 1900s, along the world's longest international border—the strip of land that divides Canada from United States—emigrating U.S. doctors trickled into Canada through dozens of border entry ports.

Scribbling on a government immigration landing document called Form 30 that recorded their personal information and reason for moving north, when asked for their occupation the newcomers invariably wrote, "Doctor."

Some were medical doctors (MDs) or general practitioners (GPs) and some were doctors of osteopathy who were later to be referred as "doctors of osteopathic medicine" both in the United States and Canada. The osteopaths did not have a traditional medical degree but graduated in osteopathy with a DO (Doctor of Osteopathy) degree from the then-fledgling American School of Osteopathy in Kirksville, Missouri, founded by Andrew Taylor Still, the medical doctor who pioneered osteopathy in 1874.

Other crossing osteopathic doctors did not attend the Kirksville school but attended other osteopathy schools that later opened to capitalize on the new medicine trend.

The Demand for Osteopathic Treatments

Ever since Canada's first osteopaths set up shop, Canadian media—and social media since the 1990s—have been covering stories on Canadians turning to the newfangled medical technology called osteopathy brought over by DOs from south of the border. Everywhere the DOs settled, residents embraced osteopathy treatments wholeheartedly because it was helping dissolve their pains and discomforts and in many cases, resolved longstanding medical problems.

Up to this day, the popularity of this natural medicine, called osteopathy, is unquestioned. The following is a fairly modern-day example.

Landing in New Brunswick from England in 1980 with her husband and her manual osteopathic skills in tow, Pierrette Richer set up shop in that maritime province. Thirty years later, in 2015, she estimated that she and the sixteen members of the Association of Osteopaths of New Brunswick have a combined patient list of more than 35,000.

Richer, who would succeed the first leader of the young osteopathy group, learned early that she didn't need to advertise her services in the Yellow Pages (in fact, she was told by the health authorities she wasn't allowed to do so). However, she found out that word had spread quickly in the northern New Brunswick city of Ville de Miramichi where she had settled, that her osteopathic manual skills were helping plenty of people overcome stubborn medical issues.

A London, Ontario – based sociologist who has delved deeply in the history of Canadian osteopathy notes that osteopaths enjoyed high stature and status in communities in the 1920s. She wrote recently that the "[o]steopaths' patient base was strong and growing, and they had achieved a general level of acceptance, especially in urban areas."[3]

In fact, public demand for osteopathic and other alternate medical treatments has been generally high and spiked to an unprecedented level in the 1970s and onwards as a result of the holistic health movement that incubated and flourished in California and crossed quickly north of the 49th parallel to Canada.

Between 1900 and 1950, Canadians were very practically minded when they faced the scourge of major diseases; they made deliberate personal decisions to seek out alternate healers—wherever the practitioners were located—when medical doctors were unable to help them.[4]

Canadians have also been quick and willing to be part of new approaches to health betterment—so much so that Hans Baer, a researcher who specializes in the politics of alternative therapies, described the changes as part of "a medical revitalization movement" that "challenged the bureaucratic, high tech and iatrogenic aspects of conventional medicine or what medical anthropologists call biomedicine."[5]

Internationally, osteopathy gained tremendous followers ranging from ordinary citizens to members of the elite. According to Quebec's Educational Institute of Osteopathy, John D. Rockefeller, Henry A. Kissinger, U.S. presidents Theodore Roosevelt, Dwight D. Eisenhower, and John F. Kennedy reportedly attributed increased wellness to osteopathic treatments.[6]

For many decades, the British Royal Family has sought the services of osteopaths. The Duke of Connaught and Princess Patricia of Connaught (a great granddaughter of Queen Victoria), "committed their physical welfare to osteopaths," according to N.J. Neilson, president of the Ontario Academy of Osteopathy in 1935.[7]

Today, Princess Anne, invested by Queen Elizabeth II as the current Princess Royal in the British Royal Family, is a Patron of the British School of Osteopathy, one of the top manual osteopathic training institutions in Western Europe.[8]

Notably, Lord Noel-Buxton, a famous British politician during the 1920s, lauded osteopathy for curing his ailment when orthodox medicine had failed.[9]

In the United Kingdom, according to a 1995 survey, 40 per cent of 760 general medical practices provided access to millions of osteopathy and other complementary therapies, which are considered the "acceptable face of complementary medicine." Between 1977 and 1997, there has been "an explosion in the public use and the professional and commercial development of complementary health care," an observer noted. "This movement has developed organically in the U.K., facilitated by [the] common law and the hands-off approach of the Conservative Government, in line with its philosophy of reliance on market forces."[10]

Iconic Canadian athletes and their recovery from mishaps through the use of osteopathy have generated positive publicity for the osteopathic profession. Former Canadian Olympic diver and 1997 World Cup tower champion Myriam Boileau, for instance, credited globetrotting osteopath Guy Voyer for saving her career after suffering for 15 months from a back injury.[11] Wendel Clark, a professional ice hockey winger who had been a three-time captain of the Toronto Maple Leafs, went to a London osteopath in 1987 after suffering a series of back and shoulder injuries. He told the media that without the help of a British osteopath, he wouldn't have been able to rejoin the team.[12]

A Wake-Up Call—Recognition of DO Qualification Refused

Early last century, the first wave of emigrating doctors of osteopathy settled along the southern parts of British Columbia in the west to New Brunswick in the east (Newfoundland and Labrador were not part of Canada until 1949). As word spread widely in the United States that Canada was a new frontier for practitioners, U.S.-based osteopaths began to trickle across the border in increasing numbers.

In Ontario, for example, during the second decade of the 20th century, there were 20 "qualified osteopaths" on the membership roster of the Toronto Association of Osteopathic Physicians, another 86 on the Ontario Osteopathic Association's roster, and 19 more members in the Toronto Osteopathic Association.[13] Research done by a newspaper reporter in1980 showed there were only 58—37 in Ontario—and their average age was 71.[14]

The first osteopath to settle in New Brunswick was during the early 1920s.[15] In British Columbia, the first three osteopathic doctors arrived around 1909.[16] In Manitoba, the first DO arrived in 1899.[17] The first osteopath to take up residence in Quebec was at the turn of the 20th century. By 1911, the number grew to five.[18]

It didn't take long for these new residents to learn that they had to contend not only with harsh winters but also with something far more formidable: the Canadian provincial and territorial governments, in consultation with the powerful provincial (officially referred to as colleges of physicians and surgeons) and territorial (health councils in the territories) regulatory colleges limited their scope of practice. In other words, they weren't generally allowed to practise medicine in the traditional sense of the word, and were prohibited from using the title "Doctor."

In Ontario, the destination of choice for most DOs, the College of Physicians and Surgeons of Ontario (CPSO) refused them a certificate of registration to practise medicine. Some jurisdictions reluctantly yielded to the DOs' demands, but with conditions. In Quebec, for example, the medical doctors agreed with the Legislative Assembly in 1922 and 1927 to amend the Medical Practice Act to help slightly improve the DOs' practice conditions but full-scale legislative recognition was never granted.[19]

The Western provinces were a little more accepting. Saskatchewan passed the *Osteopathy Act* in 1913 and with that, the province held the distinction of having the first official board for registration and examination of osteopaths outside the United States. This distinction was short-lived, however, when it was repealed—the *Drugless Practitioners Act* of 1917 replaced it.[20] The pendulum then swung the other way when the *Osteopathic Practice Act* of 1944 was enacted, only to be taken off the law books yet again this century.

The Challenge of 'Unqualified' Osteopaths

The doctors of osteopathy who came to Canada early in the 20th century graduated from two types of U.S. osteopathic training institutions. There were those schools recognized by the American Osteopathic Association (AOA), and then there were those that were believed to be fly-by-night operators—with comparatively lower educational standards—intent on capitalizing on osteopathy (which in the 1870s represented a new form of medicine).

Canadian provincial governments and their colleges of physicians and surgeons (the medical regulatory authorities) were acutely aware of the dichotomous quality of American osteopathic education. This reality would later stymie the efforts of Ontario osteopathy groups to garner favourable commentary from the 1917 provincial inquiry into medical education. The head of the inquiry, Mr. Justice Frank Hodgins, was quick to observe that while some U.S. osteopathic schools reached a desirable standard with the AMA, as a whole, the schools were not producing graduates of a similar calibre due to the fledging nature of the profession.[21]

Feeling threatened by the inflow of seemingly under-qualified upstarts, the Toronto Association of Osteopathic Physicians pushed back. It placed an advertisement in the 1916 annual edition of the *Bell Company Directory* to distance themselves from these U.S. graduates.

"In the absence of legislation," the notice read, "regulating the practice of osteopathy, and the consequent invasion of Ontario by hosts of unqualified persons calling themselves osteopaths, the Toronto Association of Osteopathic Physicians publishes [a] list of qualified osteopaths who are now [August 1, 1916] practising in the city . . . ." The association also pointed out that "all graduates of colleges [are] now requiring for graduation a minimum course of three years, each of nine months actual attendance and work." The ad listed the names of its 20 members.

Legislative 'Discouragement' a Bugaboo for Canadian Osteopathic Practice

Canadian-based osteopathic doctors who were trained in the United States have been, from day one, impassioned soldiers in their march for equal status with medical doctors who had long before secured title and practice rights protection under provincial and territorial laws.

Because of the pathway along which conventional medicine developed—from the beginning of formal training of doctors in Italian universities in 1220 to proving the germ theory of disease from the mid-16th century to current advancements in chemistry, genetics, and lab technology—medical doctors became the first health professionals to secure the legal title of "Doctor."[22]

With it, medical doctors enjoyed the rights, privileges and power to practise the full scope of medical practice from diagnosing and treating diseases to performing surgery. Needless to say, they guarded these benefits with great determination.

So, from the late 1800s, Canadian medical doctors have enjoyed a strong dominative status and worked hard to effectively shut out scores of alternate and complementary medicine groups, including osteopathy, from securing regulatory status.

This power was exercised and maintained through the colleges of physicians and surgeons which the provincial governments created through legislation. Administered largely by medical doctors, these organizations have had a vested interest in preventing other medical practitioners from becoming "legitimate medicine," And, for a long time, the high trust level it developed with the governments of all political stripes further strengthened their massive capacity to have a say in excluding others from being regulated for a long time.[23]

So when governments pass laws that discourage the advancement of a health profession group (especially when they reduce the scope of practice of its practitioners), it may be assumed, from a political standpoint, that the government has been more influenced in their decision by more powerful, entrenched groups than by those who are advocating for a higher legislative standing.

A great deal of the history of Canadian osteopathy—and kindred professions such as naturopathy, traditional Chinese medicine, acupuncture and chiropractic—is riddled with examples of such government policies that are traceable to the lobbying efforts of the provincial medical regulatory authorities.

Conversely, when laws, such as Registration Acts, or amendments to medical statutes, are enacted that bestow a wider scope of practice and even regulatory status to those health professions that were previously unregulated, they encourage the development of the profession.

B.C. Osteopathic Doctors and Their Case of Being 'More Discouraged Than Encouraged'

The first doctors of osteopathic medicine who arrived in Canada's most westernmost province were not immune to the demoralizing effect of being rejected by the government when they sought regulation to practise osteopathic medicine on the same basis as medical doctors.

At the turn of the 20th century when the first three osteopaths opened up their practice, medical doctors had strong reservations about the medicine practised by the newcomers. The doctors therefore descended on their provincial parliamentary members urging them to introduce a bill "to nullify osteopathic practice.[24]

But the residents of the province who reaped benefits from the new medical therapy became incensed by the actions of the medical doctors and loudly made their views known to the politicians. The medical doctors, in response, withdrew their bill.

Some heartening developments followed. In 1909, the B.C. provincial government, after consulting the College of Physicians and Surgeons of British Columbia, amended the *Medical Act* to allow osteopaths to take medical practitioner candidate examinations. Instead of being examined on medicine and therapeutics, they had to write a paper on the principles and practice of osteopathy.

This concession allowed osteopathic physicians to sign birth and death certificates, gave them access to hospitals, and allowed them to manage narcotics usage. In other words, osteopathic physicians were given a wider slate of practice rights but were not allowed to perform surgery, according to a medical historian and former dean of medicine at the University of Toronto.[25]

Later in the 20th century, the osteopaths became disheartened when those privileges were withdrawn. During and after the 1930s, "relations with the medical profession gradually deteriorated."

Today, osteopathic physicians must register with the College of Physicians and Surgeons of British Columbia in order to practice in the province. The college has already changed its policies to align with the agreement it signed in 2003 with other provinces and the territories to introduce a "National Standard" for medical licensure. This agreement was developed by the Federation of Medical Regulatory Authorities of Canada.

Manitoba Osteopathic Doctors and Their Case of Being 'More Discouraged Than Encouraged'

Following the founding of the Manitoba Osteopathic Association in 1913 with six members, the group went to the wall a year later when they unsuccessfully attempted to secure licensing legislation.

Undaunted, the osteopathic physicians and the chiropractors began advertising their services widely and lobbied the politicians intensively. They ". . . offered their services regularly and seldom with repercussion . . . and . . . consistently organized and brought forth bills with the intention of broadening their practices."[26]

In 1921, they tried again unsuccessfully to secure legislation to legitimize osteopathic medical practice so that they would be on par with medical doctors. As has been the case with the medical profession in other provinces, Manitoba's medical doctors "rallied around the notion that alternative practitioners, or 'quacks', posed a threat to public health" during the infancy period of osteopathy and chiropractic in Canada. "The Manitoba medical profession, undeniably, perceived alternative medicine as an irritation, an outrage, and perhaps even to a lesser extent as competition."[27]

For another two decades, the tremendous political power of the medical doctors were brought to bear in dampening any legislative initiatives by the politicians to grant licensure to osteopathic practitioners in Manitoba.

Things have changed since. Today, section 11(1)(b) of Manitoba's *Medical Act*, has created an "educational register" for all medical graduates. This allows U.S. osteopathic college graduates to take part in post-graduate training programs that are supervised by medical staff. This additional training and related examinations—such as those from the Medical Council of Canada—are part of the required qualifications outlined in Manitoba's *Regulation 25/2003* to meet registration requirements for an osteopathic physician's licence. The Manitoba College of Physicians and Surgeons has also put in place "a screening process" for graduates of "other medical schools."

The Manitoba College of Physicians and Surgeons has agreed in principle, along with other provinces and the territories, to the introduction of a "National Standard" for licensure.

Quebec Osteopathic Doctors and Their Case of Being 'More Discouraged Than Encouraged'

The osteopathic physicians in "La belle province" did not escape the dispiriting effects of being turned down repeatedly by their provincial government for regulation that would give their osteopathic physicians a licence to practice.

Between 1913 and 1927, they tried three times, unsuccessfully, to sponsor bills that would authorize them to practise medicine with the province's blessings. On one of those occasions, the National Assembly in Quebec (at that time called the Legislative Assembly), rejected a 1919 piece of proposed legislation sponsored by the osteopathic physicians' association, despite an accompanying 2,500-citizen petition.[28] Later, however, the Assembly lifted the spirits of the osteopaths by passing some amendments to the *Medical Practice Act* "to improve [their] practice conditions."[29]

In the early 1930s, the prospects of attaining further status became somewhat better when a bill to grant licensure for members of the Quebec Association of Osteopathic Physicians, received a Second Reading in the Legislative Assembly. The osteopathic medical community naturally savoured the moment.

Not too long after, however, the association, ironically, pulled its support of the bill that would advance its cause. It did so under duress: its action was in exchange for the medical doctors' withdrawal of charges brought against several osteopathic physicians in 1935 for allegedly practising medicine. The medical doctors thus effectively halted the original bill just before the Third Reading in parliament.

Today, U.S.-trained osteopathic physicians would be recognized by Quebec's medical regulatory body as a result of a "National Standard" for medical licensure adopted by the province. The standard, developed by the Federation of Medical Regulatory Authorities of Canada, of which Quebec is a member, requires osteopathic doctors to pass the MCCQE Parts 1 and 2 examinations (set by the Medical Council of Canada) and successfully complete a residency.

However, the medical register of the Collège des médecins du Québec has no record of medical doctors practising osteopathy.

Saskatchewan Osteopathic Doctors and Their Case of Being 'More Discouraged Than Encouraged'

The historical experience of osteopathic physicians who practised in the "Land of Rapeseed and Honey"—a nickname for the province of Saskatchewan—illustrates how a seemingly encouraging legislative body can change its collective mind and display unanticipated discouraging behaviour toward the same group.

Osteopathic medical professionals in Saskatchewan went through ups and downs from being a health profession with high recognition status to one where there was a large withdrawal of official recognition. In 1944, Saskatchewan enacted the *Osteopathic Practice Act* to grant U.S.-trained doctors of osteopathic medicine almost full medical rights: they were allowed to order X-rays, and write prescriptions but they were not allowed to perform surgery.[30]

However, from May 26, 2005, onwards, they no longer were able to carry on their then six-decade old tradition. This game-changer came about when the NDP government of Lorne Calvert introduced Bill No. 116 for First Reading in the Legislative Assembly (the *Osteopathic Practice Repeal Act*) on April 27, 2005.

The rationales that the then Health Minister John Nilson outlined for sending the osteopaths into near oblivion were that "the Act is obsolete; and . . . there are currently no osteopathic physicians practising in Saskatchewan nor have there been for many years."[31]

As to the lack of practitioners in Saskatchewan at that time, the health minister was correct. Regina, Alta. – based Dr. Anna Northup and Dr. Doris Tanner, the last two osteopathic physicians in the province, had died many years earlier -- Dr. Northup in 1977 and Dr. Tanner shortly thereafter. Accompanying Dr. Northup's death, after 46 years of practice, was the simultaneous demise of the Saskatchewan Society of Osteopathic Physicians of which she was its first president.[32]

To further rationalize his decision, Nilson also explained that osteopathic medical training in the United States had changed over the years to include a broader scope of practice. "Consequently a Canadian-trained osteopath would not likely be eligible for licensure under the current Act. Graduates from an American program could potentially be licensed in Saskatchewan, but they would be unable to practise to the full scope of their education," he told parliamentarians.

"The repeal of the Act will not prevent an osteopath from establishing practice in the province as long as they do not engage in any treatment that encroaches on the scope of practice of any other regulated professionals," he added.

That modern-day blow to Saskatchewan's osteopathic physicians was nothing new, in fact. In 1913, the government of the day enacted the *Osteopathic Act* paving the way for osteopaths to obtain a license to practise. Practise, the osteopaths did, but only for three years.

With the passing of a new law in 1917—the *Drugless Practitioners Act* (DPA, for short)—the provincial government pulled the rug from under the osteopathic physicians, and they suddenly had a new status: that of being a "drugless practitioner."[33]

How Ontario Osteopaths Generally Fought and Kept Their Heads Above Water—An Overview

Ontario was the scene of the one of the most widely known open confrontations between osteopaths and the traditional medical establishment. In 1900, two years after the province's first osteopathic doctor arrived in town, he had to go to court to defend his professional honour.

Robert B. Henderson, of St. Marys, Ontario, was charged by the College of Physicians and Surgeons of Ontario for practising medicine without a licence after opening his practice in the year he arrived.[34]

(The court ruled in the college's favour, but the conviction was later quashed by Judge Morson in a March 1910 ruling.)[35]

Many medical historians and political analysts have demonstrated in their research that during the 20th century, the medical establishment had been successful in influencing the shape of legislation that protected its strong position throughout that time.

Its power over the politicians was evident when osteopath groups approached the Ontario government with requests for better consideration of their cause. A 1980 newspaper report on the reaction of the Ontario regulatory authorities to osteopaths revealed a merry-go-round-type scenario:

According to Dr. H.W. Henderson, the Deputy Registrar of the college, osteopathic doctors weren't licensed to practise medicine in Ontario because "there are no provisions under Ontario legislation for recognizing osteopathy." The legislation, he said, was the responsibility of the Ministry of Health, and if the law was going to change, the Ministry of Health would have to do it.

The Ministry of Health, in turn, said it had given the responsibility to the College of Physicians and Surgeons, and the college had the authority to set the standards for medical training. "It is not policy to have osteopaths practising medicine in Ontario," a Ministry of Health spokesman said. "It's a college decision."[36]

Around the same time, Eugene Forsey, a Canadian constitution expert, had a similar experience. As chairperson of the London, Ontario –based Canadian Osteopathic Aid Society (a lay group that championed osteopathic health care), he wrote to the media about his frustration: "When we have asked the Government for action [to allow osteopathic physicians to practise on the same basis as other physicians] they have replied that it is a matter for the College of Physicians and Surgeons of

Ontario. When we have asked the College of Physicians and Surgeons, they have replied that it is a matter for the Government."[37]

**

As noted earlier, during the 1920s osteopaths made "significant strides towards achieving professional status."[38] Whatever progress they made, however, was pockmarked by a wholesale condemnation of what osteopaths stood for. During that period, "the medical profession refused to accept them as colleagues and professed to find them a threat to the health of the public. They felt that such people should be prohibited entirely from practising, unless they had also completed an orthodox medical education.[39]

In Ontario, the more influential members of the medical community denounced osteopathy in no uncertain terms. An associate professor of clinical medicine at the University of Toronto, reflected the typical physician's view of osteopaths in the 1920s, by describing them as part of a group of "irregular practitioners" and adherents of "cults on this continent" who should be given "no special favours" and insisted that there must be "one portal of entry into the medical profession [that is, through the Medical Council examinations]."[40]

Referring specifically to chiropractors and osteopaths, the associate professor called them "an enormous financial burden . . . by the support of this army of self-styled doctors."[41] A present-day observer described the medical doctors' perceptions this way: "Organized medicine's strongest reactions were reserved for osteopaths and chiropractors."[42]

The osteopathic colleges that trained the osteopaths did not escape criticism, either: "The eight osteopathic schools [in the early 1910s] reeked with commercialism. Their catalogues are a mass of hysterical exaggerations alike of the earning and the curative power of osteopathy, etc."[43]

Undauntedly, the osteopathic community fired back with torrents of words against the medical mainstream establishment. And when Ontario osteopaths held meetings they expressed their frustration at being unable to match the political power of the medical doctors.

In their endless struggles, Ontario-based osteopathic doctors found an ally outside their ranks: Toronto's largest newspaper, *The Toronto Daily Star*, which later evolved into *The Toronto Star*. A number of headlines on its Op-Ed pages were clearly supportive: "Ontario's Injustice Toward Osteopaths Rooted in the Past,"[44] and "Give Osteopaths a Break,"[45] and "Osteopathy Too Valuable to be Lost."[46]

A Close Look at the Period from 1900 through the 1920s

In 1916, Justice Frank Hodgins in his provincial inquiry into the state of medical education in Ontario learned that three provinces—Alberta, Saskatchewan and British Columbia—"provided for the admission of osteopaths to practise" in the early decades of the 20th century.[47]

Specifically, between 1906 and 1916, Alberta-based osteopathic doctors who had the same basic education as an ordinary medical student and possessed a graduation diploma from an American Osteopathic Association-recognized school of osteopathy, were allowed to practise if they passed certain examinations. These were regular medical examinations, except in surgery and medicine. For surgery, the osteopath candidate was tested on surgical diagnosis and the conduct of minor operations; and for medicine, he or she was examined in the theory and practice of osteopathy.

In Ontario, however, osteopathic doctors were not particularly optimistic about the future, due to the different issues and various political scenarios facing them. Also, they had to deal with more "downs" than "ups."

In 1910, Bill 47, a bill sponsored by Ontario MPP Dr. Jamieson for the registration and regulation of osteopaths as well as to "Incorporate the Osteopathic College of Ontario" later led to the appointment of a legislative committee to study the bill's measures which "were almost identical and followed the *Medical Act*."[48]

The hearings were especially tense. A Toronto Star reporter described the discussions of several meetings as "warm and strenuous." During one of them, committee member W.R. McNaught strongly pushed for osteopaths to go back to school. He called for osteopaths to do a three-year course in a school of osteopathy that was approved by both the Medical Council of Canada and Ontario's Lieutenant-Governor—irrespective of their many years of training they had to qualify for the doctor of osteopathy degree in the United States.[49]

McNaught also pushed for a new clause to prescribe that osteopaths pass the primary and final examinations of the Medical Council "with a paper on osteopathy substituted for the usual paper on *materia medica*," and that January 1, 1912 be the deadline for osteopaths without a diploma to obtain certification from a recognized U.S. osteopathic college in order to practise. The original clause had called for osteopaths to have five years of practice experience to be eligible to treat patients.

The College of Physicians and Surgeons participated in the hearings. In its presentation to the committee, it "pushed to keep osteopathy on an inferior footing by preventing osteopaths from prescribing drugs or performing surgery."[50]

The legislative committee eventually rejected the bill.

In response to continuing public pressure for osteopaths and other alternate health professions to be considered for regulation, and the continuing opposition by the College of Physicians and Surgeons of Ontario against the many new health-care therapies that were becoming available to residents, the provincial government appointed a royal commission headed by Mr. Justice Frank Hodgins on September 29, 1915, to review the osteopaths' case as part of a larger investigation on medical education.

Justice Hodgins was mandated to report on the "present positions, status and practice of osteopaths, dentists, nurses, opticians, optometrists, chiropractors, Christian scientists, or others practising or professing medicine.[51]

Because "medicine" was not defined properly in the Ontario *Medical Act* of 1914, the commissioner provided a context for his study, defining medicine as:

> *any science, plan, method or system with or without the use of drugs or appliances, and whether now deemed to be included therein or not, for diagnosing , prescribing for preventing, alleviating, treating or curing human disorders, illnesses, diseases, ailments, pains, wounds, suffering, injury or deformity affecting the human body or any part thereof or its physical condition, or believed or imagined so to do, including midwifery, and any treatment prescribed advised, intended or professing immediately or ultimately to benefit the patient.*

After listening to the osteopathic groups at hearings and reviewing their written briefs, Hodgins recommended that Ontario should not follow Saskatchewan, Alberta and British Columbia's models in registering osteopaths. One of his main reasons was that he believed Ontario's medical education and equipment standards were higher than those of the western provinces.

He also concluded that Ontario osteopaths faced a major issue. "[There is] the want of cohesion among those practising osteopathy in Ontario, and the consequent absence of any serious attempt to establish and maintain a high standard of attainment and practice," the Commissioner wrote in his final report.[52]

But the key rationale he provided for disallowing parity of osteopathic doctors with medical doctors was his sense that the body of osteopathic knowledge was still in a "state of transition."[53]

Based mainly on the findings and recommendations of the Hodgins inquiry as well as giving in to pressure from the powerful College of Physicians and Surgeons of Ontario, the Ontario government passed, in 1925, the *Drugless Practitioners Act* (DPA).

The first set of regulations released under the Act in the fall of 1926 assigned osteopathic doctors to one of five drugless practitioner classifications (Drugless practitioners are those who practise "the treatment of any ailment, disease, both defect or disability of the human body by manipulation, adjustment, manual or electro-therapy or by any similar method."[54]). The osteopath classification required the osteopathic physicians to follow a "specified educational program and pass a Board [of Regents]–administered licensing examination."[55]

The DPA took effect at an interesting time—during the Roaring Twenties. This was a period marked by unprecedented cultural and economic changes when jazz music reach new heights and people felt more prosperous. But osteopathic physicians felt abandoned, and most had no motivation to continue to pursue their goal to obtain proper recognition of their talent. In dire frustration, they cried discrimination. Most Ontario-based osteopaths returned to the United States; some went west where the provincial governments and the physicians and surgeons' colleges were relatively more welcoming.

The 1930s—The Great Depression Years

In the decades following the proclamation of drugless practitioners laws in other jurisdictions, (for example, Saskatchewan's *Drugless Practitioners Act* of 1928-29[56]), the provincial regulatory and licensing colleges of physicians and surgeons, along with the federal and provincial governments, were criticized heavily by Canadian and American osteopathy leaders for alleged favouritism. That is, due to their close ties to the politicians, the medical regulatory colleges representing medical doctors, were able to unduly influence public policy to protect their privileges.

Addressing the 35th annual convention of the Ontario Academy of Osteopathy in 1937 at the King Edward Hotel in Toronto, the visiting dean of the Chicago-based College of Osteopathy, Richard Bain, expressed his dismay with the attitude of Canada's medical doctors. "The medical profession is more antagonistic than ever to the osteopaths," declared McBain, a former resident of Oakville, Ontario.[57]

A month earlier, Hubert Pocock, a leading light in the Canadian professional osteopathic community, applauded Ontario's decision to give osteopaths the right to treat workers under the *Workers' Compensation Act*, and assured medical doctors that "it won't jeopardize the medical man because our work is not in his sphere." And he lambasted the medical regulatory college because it "has done everything in its power to interfere with the osteopathic profession receiving its due rights."[58]

In 1933, the Ontario Legislature considered a bill that would regulate the practice of osteopathy and set out qualifications for practitioners. It was referred to a standing committee headed by Minister of Mines Charles McCrea. The bill sought to empower osteopaths "to use any prefix or affix describing or referring to any professional status or degree which the osteopath possesses, such as doctor of osteopathy or osteopathic physician," and to set up a board of registrars who would decide whether an osteopath is qualified or not to practise.[59]

This bill, which would have conferred professional status for both osteopaths and homeopaths, went nowhere. On Monday, April 10, 1933, a legal bills committee chaired by Minister McCrea, rejected it. Said the minister: "There is no doubt great benefits [would be bestowed] . . . on sufferers by osteopathy. [But] this bill goes too far and we will have to work out some means for the advantage and protection of the public."[60]

During the 1930s, the college appointed a two-inspector team (a faculty member from the University of Toronto's faculty of medicine and one from Queen's University) to go on a fact-finding trip to the United States to research osteopathic training institutions. They returned to Toronto delivering an unflattering report to the college registrar about American osteopathic training.

But Toronto osteopaths retorted the college's claim and told Dr. J.M. Robb, Ontario's minister of health in 1934, that the doctors visited only one classroom during their two-and-a-half hour visit to the longest established osteopathic college in the United States. They also alleged the two Canadian doctors had attended no clinics, heard no lectures, and made no check-ups on laboratory findings.[61]

The 1940s—The Second World War Years

The anger and frustration of osteopaths were even more vehement during the Second World War. Because medical personnel, particularly medical doctors, were in great shortage in taking care of wounded Canadian soldiers, the professional osteopathic community urged the federal government to utilize osteopaths to help.

Instead, many osteopathic physicians were being drafted into the army as combat soldiers, much to the chagrin of the president of the York County Osteopathic Association in Ontario. He wrote to the editor of a newspaper, saying: "I wish to make public protest against the unfair and incomplete manner in which our war effort is being carried out with respect to health services both for the fighting forces and for civilian workers."[62] (Ironically, south of the border, the U.S. Army Forces widely utilized the services of osteopathic doctors.)

Canadian soldiers found great comfort and relief with osteopathic treatments. A survey of some 6,000 men in the Canadian armed services by the Canadian Osteopathic Association revealed that the soldiers actively sought—and paid for out of their own pockets—osteopathic physicians' help "to obtain relief they were unable to get from army medical personnel," declared George A. De Jardine, president of the Canadian Osteopathic Association (COA), in a brief to the House of Commons' Social Security committee in 1943.[63]

Why did unwounded but worn-out Canadian soldiers prefer osteopathic doctors?

The support for and benefits of osteopathic manual manipulative techniques by soldiers were clearly explained by a Chicago-based osteopathic doctor: "There is so much wear and tear on a soldier's physical mechanism in a half-hour ride in a speeding tank or armoured car as there was in a whole day's trench-digging or marching," the doctor said. "Because of that there is a rapidly growing need in armies for physicians [like osteopaths] to correct disturbed body mechanics with manipulative therapeutics."[64]

A Small Victory for Ontario Osteopaths After the Second World War

Seven years after the war ended in 1945, Premier Leslie Frost and the Progressive Conservative government of Ontario conceded to the osteopaths following constant lobbying by the Ontario Osteopathic Association. Through an Order-in-Council, issued by Lieutenant–Governor Louis O. Breithaupt, Ontario's osteopaths—and chiropractors—were allowed to create a board for self-rule, called the Board of Osteopathic Practitioners.

A governing board meant that its members acquired the power to discipline their members and monitor the qualifications of their members.

This breakthrough was described by *The Toronto Star*:

The 20-year battle by Ontario osteopaths for the right to govern, license and examine members of their profession ended in victory today [Nov. 6, 1952] with the announcement by the provincial government that a board of directors of osteopathy has been established.[65] For the past 26 years osteopaths have been lumped in with physiotherapists, chiropractors and massage [therapists] under the all-embracing Drugless Practitioners Act, *and governed by a common board of regents.[66]*

Although this was a far cry from being supervised by the Board of Regents established under the *Drugless Practitioners Act* of 1925, it did not meet their expectations regarding broader practice rights. They were still not allowed provide the full range of medical care that included authorization to order X-rays, write prescriptions, or do surgery. In other words, they were still restricted to doing spinal manipulations.

This was clearly not the kind of regulation befitting their skill levels in medicine. While some osteopaths saw the new development as being progress, it was largely perceived to be a continuation of the exclusionary tactics by both the government and the medical regulatory college.

Public relations director of the Ontario Osteopathic Association was unflinching in his criticism: The board was established primarily "to ease its [the government's] administrative headaches. We cannot regard it as an acknowledgement by the government of the growing stature of the profession in the eyes of the public."[67]

(Members of the first Ontario Osteopathic Association board were: Douglas Firth representing the Ontario Osteopathic Association (chair); J.R.F McVity (vice-chair); D.G.A Campbell (secretary/treasurer); Ray Linnen of Ottawa (member); Norman Burbidge of Guelph (member); and a ministry of health representative.)

The Ontario government disbanded the board in the 1980s.

The Decades of the 1960s and 1970s

The political mood in the mid-20th century and beyond was one of heightened awareness of the need for greater public accountability among health-care professionals. This was not surprising given the increasing media reports of patients complaining about non-conventional health practitioners and not having a proper avenue to air their complaints and obtain redress.

At the same time, the government was also concerned about strengthening the civil rights of Ontario residents as part of its desire to create a more equal and just society.

Also fuelling the need for changes in the health-care system was provincial and territorial governments' obligation to adhere to federal government guidelines and standards for funding their universal health insurance systems.

To address these broad problems, in late 1966 the Ontario government appointed Torontonian and businessman I.R. Dowie to head a three-person commission, called the Committee on the Healing Arts (an investigative group similar to the 1917 Hodgins Royal Commission on medical education) to examine the health professions system and make recommendations on their future regulation and educational requirements. The committee's overall mandate was to "enquire into and report on all matters relating to the education and regulation relevant to the practice of the healing arts."[68]

Ontario had also set up a royal commission, a little earlier, to study and make recommendations on reforms to better protect individual rights in provincial law. This commission was headed by James McRuer, the Chief Justice of Ontario when the federal government passed the *Canadian Bill of Rights* in 1960. An important theme underlying the 1968 McRuer report and the 1970 healing arts study was the call for more openness in bureaucratic processes. This was seen as appearing to challenge the power of entrenched medical practitioner groups in Ontario, such as medical doctors and dentists.

The healing arts inquiry strongly argued for halting "the proliferation of professions" by preventing other health professions from using the "doctor title" behind their members' name. At the same time, however, it advocated the need for a more balanced view of what it called "vulnerable interests, referring to other provider groups that have been excluded from mainstream medical practice, like the osteopaths, for example, for a long time.[69]

In opening up the health-care market to professionals other than those few groups having a monopolistic share of the health-care provider market, some economists who had been advocating for reduced government intervention in the market, agreed with the inquiry's findings. They suggested opening up the system so that health practitioner groups could have a chance to practise with the full privileges of being self-governed.[70]

Like other whole-body healing arts groups, such as the Ontario Naturopathic Association representing naturopathic medicine practitioners, the Ontario Osteopathic Association submitted a brief recommending that osteopathic medicine be brought under the umbrella of the College of Physicians and Surgeons of Ontario in order to bring it into the mainstream of medical care.

With a counter-proposal, the College of Physicians and Surgeons of Ontario (CPSO) recommended that the "non-medical" professions should treat only patients referred to them by medical doctors. Chiding the CPSO, University of Toronto professor Horace Krever (a member of the healing arts inquiry board and later a judge in Ontario's Court of Appeal), described the college's ideas as having the potential effect of putting "all chiropractors, osteopaths and other non-medical healers out of business in Ontario."

When the Committee on Healing Arts finally wrapped up its findings and presented its recommendations in 1970, however, it essentially followed in the footsteps of its counterpart investigating group—the Hodgins Royal Commission—more than half a century earlier. Referring to the osteopaths, the committee said it was not happy with the quality of their education. Interestingly, the committee's chairman, I.R. Dowie, reportedly told the media that it was difficult for medical doctors and osteopaths to be objective in appraising each other's education.[71]

Following up on the findings and recommendations of the Dowie inquiry, the Conservative government, under Premier William Davis, introduced draft legislation for the *Health Disciplines Act* (HDA).

While the main thrust of the HDA was to regulate five health professions (dentistry, medicine, nursing, optometry and pharmacy), it proposed, among other things, a Health Practitioners Registration Council to govern the professional affairs of groups of healers such as osteopaths and speech therapists.[72]

The rationale for placing osteopaths under the proposed council, along with other non-medical health practitioners, was that there were too few osteopaths in Ontario at that time—in fact, only a dozen or so.

Following meetings between the osteopathic association and the ministry of health, S. W. Martin, the then deputy minister of health, informed the osteopaths in a letter that any changes to their status would have to be based on the College of Physicians and Surgeons of Ontario's recommendation equating osteopaths' training and qualifications with those of medical doctors.

The college eventually decided to disallow the osteopaths a licence to practise medicine.

Soon after the latest rejection by the medical regulator, *The Toronto Star*, a long-time supporter for osteopaths gaining full practice rights, described the osteopaths' plight in an editorial as "getting an official run around from the provincial government" and declared that "to leave the fate of the profession in the hands of a rival professional body is wholly unjust."[73]

Four years earlier, the paper had pummelled the regulatory powers that be in an editorial denouncing the "long battle by medical men against them."[74]

With this latest blow, the osteopaths in Ontario were once again stymied in their bid for regulation. In an effort to move forward, the osteopathic association thought of another strategy: Why not establish a chair of osteopathy at an Ontario university?[75]

The osteopaths, with the support of the Canadian Osteopathic Association, in concert with Michigan State University's College of Osteopathic Medicine, proposed to the Ministry of Training, Colleges and Universities, that a college of osteopathic medicine be set up in Sarnia's Lambton College.[76] The ministry turned down the proposal. The government's decision also put the nail in the coffin of a dream that Robert H. Henderson, Ontario's first osteopath, told a newspaper in 1906: "I think that the day may come in Canada when there may be a chair of osteopathy in our university here [in Toronto]."[77]

In Quebec in the 1970s, the members – estimated to be fewer than five – of the now defunct Quebec Association of Osteopathic Physicians were not prepared to practise in French, and left La belle province in a huff. In 1974, the province's Premier Robert Bourassa and his Liberal government passed the *Official Language Act* (Bill 22), making French the official language of Quebec.

Three years later, on August 26, 1977 with the enactment of Bill 101, (the French language charter), spearheaded by the Parti Québecois government of René Lévesque, the fundamental French language rights in the 1974 legislation were strengthened.

The 1980s to 1999: The Slow and Steady Rise of Osteopathic Manual Medicine

The 1980s was marked by the beginning of the Canadian movement for practitioners who were trained only in osteopathic manual practice, unlike the osteopathic practitioners who had come to Canada in the late 1800s, and had been trained in U.S. osteopathic colleges as doctors of osteopathic medicine.

Thanks to French-born Philippe Druelle, osteopathic manual practice took off with the opening, in 1981, of the first osteopathic manual school in Montreal, the Collège d'Études Ostéopathiques. Druelle later established campuses in British Columbia, Manitoba, Nova Scotia and Ontario. He also subsequently launched The Foundation for Teaching and Research in Osteopathy to promote "traditional" osteopathy."

The first graduates of the Montreal school, although just a handful, joined the estimated remaining 19 aging doctors of osteopathic medicine in Ontario (their average age in the '70s was 65), such as Victor de Jardine[78] and Douglas Firth, who had practised manipulation of the body in the previous decades. The Ontario group of 19 was estimated to be more than the combined total of all the osteopathic medicine doctors in the provinces and territories.[79]

**

The ascendancy of osteopathic manual medicine and osteopathic manual professionals in the 1980s unfolded in a unique historical period in Ontario.

For Ontarians at that time, a good working health-care system meant being able to get timely, qualified treatments from health-care practitioners as well as access to health information, a complaint system and consent to treatment.

James Ruer's report in 1978 on how to create a more equal Ontario society gave clarity and helped sensitize patients about their rights not only in health-care delivery but in all spheres of life. In their interactions with health-care providers and institutions, ordinary citizens became more empowered.

With more frequent media coverage of patient rights issues, easier interactive communications brought about by technical communications advances via the Internet, and the intense activists' work by health-care consumer advocacy groups, rights issues found a front and centre spot in public debates.

Thus, according to observers, the social and political environment around health care became ripe for further evolutionary changes.

In November 1982, Lawrence "'Larry" Grossman, Ontario's minister of health, announced the rollout of a comprehensive review of all the healing arts in an attempt to fine-tune the laws affecting the health-care professions. The review team was also asked to "devise a new structure for all legislation governing the health professions and to settle outstanding issues involving several professions."[80]

Costing $750,000, the investigation, officially called the Health Professions Legislative Review, lasted more than five years and resulted in the passing of the 1991 *Registered Health Professions Act* (RHPA), which today is touted as a model for legislating health professions across North America.

The Board of Osteopathic Practitioners of Ontario (BOPO) welcomed the move even though there were few practitioners in Ontario at that time because its scope of practice was limited to using only about 20 per cent of what they learned as U.S. osteopaths.

The value of becoming a self-regulated entity with the government's blessing through an Act of the legislature was not lost on the vying groups. Gaining licensure rights and self-governance, which means "recognition" by the government, is beautifully and succinctly described by a Ryerson University politics professor, whose book is devoted almost entirely to the review: "[what happens with becoming a self-regulated entity is that] legal procedural rights and obligations normally reserved for the judicial arm of the state's legal authority" passes over to the professional governing body.[81]

In many ways, the review created a war of words—and medical turf wars. The tensions among the groups were evident and played out in Ontario's newspapers, radio and TV news features. Much of the wrangling revolved around "the technical and legal details of the practitioners' authorized acts or procedures and scopes of practice."

The background to this battleground for competing new ideas in health-care modalities and getting the attention of the review committee had one important feature: the ethnic face of Ontario was gradually and radically transforming, thanks to Canada's more liberal immigration policy. The new immigrants from Europe, Asia and the Caribbean were accustomed to alternate and complementary medicines in their former motherlands and therefore welcomed treatments, when in Ontario, from health-care practitioners other than those from conventional doctors.

Equally important, more Ontarians were more open than ever to embracing wellness as a lifestyle to prevent disease.

It was evident, then, that the Alan Schwartz review team had to factor in this new reality and would therefore have to accommodate the demographic and lifestyle changes if it were going to do a good job. Observers, including media columnists, noted that its deliberations would have to meet societal expectations for a wider range of health-care options.

Within less than two years after the announcement of the review process, the review team decided who would be "in" and "out." It chose 39 out of the estimated 75 self-proclaimed health professional associations for further discussion and later recommended to the minister of health that 24 groups should be given self-regulatory status. Thus, the others—

more than 40 (including the interest groups representing the osteopaths, and in particular, members of the Board of Osteopathic Practitioners)— were left behind.[82]

Health critic for the New Democratic Party, MPP David Reville, who represented the Parkdale riding, summed up the feelings of some of the many groups who felt disenfranchised in the review.

Questioning Health Minister Elinor Caplan on January 26, 1989 (the day the government tabled the report not only as a report but also as draft legislation), Reville took a shot at the minister: "There are 53 health-care professions which have been left out in the cold and those people will want to come forward at some point when we see the government's law to have some things to say about all that."

The review team had hardly finished its inquiry when the Ontario Naturopathic Association president provided his two cents worth in a somewhat tongue-in-cheek fashion, saying, "The review's design is very smart. They are throwing all the professions together in the ring. There's going to be a dog fight, and the committee will act as a referee."[83]

The few doctors of osteopathic medicine in Ontario had some reason to be at least optimistic before the review was complete. On April 3, 1986, Murray Elston, the fourth health minister since Minister Grossman launched the review, announced at a news conference in Toronto that osteopaths, recognized as medical doctors in the United States, would then begin to be governed under rules by the College of Physicians and Surgeons of Ontario.

Based on that policy change, a Toronto newspaper optimistically forecasted that U.S.-trained Canadian osteopaths might return to Ontario to practise as they would no longer be governed by the *Drugless Practitioners Act*.[84]

The bottom line of the new government policy was bad news for the osteopaths: they were still not going to be able to realize their multiple-decades-old dream of being able to cross into the practice area of physicians with regard to prescribing drugs or performing surgery. Their schedule of permissible practices remained largely the same as those they had been performing under the 1925 *Drugless Practitioners Act*.

The revised scenario was they were going to be regulated by their historic adversary, the college. Moreover, those osteopaths who were going to be regulated had to have a Doctor of Osteopathy qualification issued by an accredited college of osteopathic medicine in the United States. As well, they also had to pass the MD exams like every medical graduate in every Ontario university.

In the five years of the review, the CPSO, a longstanding professional group, representing conventional medicine, thus fought a good fight in maintaining its dominance over medical expertise and knowledge.

The work of the Health Professions Legislative Review culminated in the 1991 *Regulated Health Professions Act*, or the RHPA. Its proclamation on August 1, 1992 created a landmark for the new framework on how the health professions would be self-regulated.

The changes were as unprecedented as they were far-reaching. One major change was that the family of health profession groups who were invested with self-regulatory privileges swelled: Twenty-one regulatory colleges oversaw 23 health professions within the medical and para-medical services landscape.[85]

This caused a further redistribution of power in "medicine." The dominance of a few regulated medical practitioner bodies under the 1970s *Health Disciplines Act* was reduced.

The Decade from 2000 to 2010

The first decade of the 21st century witnessed a game-changing decision by the provincial and territorial medical regulatory bodies to adopt a "National Standard" to license medical doctors and thus formalizing a pan-Canadian medical registration process.

In many jurisdictions, the main conditions that doctors of osteopathic medicine must meet to obtain full licensure is that they must be awarded a Licentiate of the Medical Council of Canada and be successful as a resident through the Royal College of Physicians and Surgeons of Canada or the College of Family Physicians of Canada.

In Ontario, for example, the CPSO adopted a policy in 2003 that "delineates the College of Physicians and Surgeons of Ontario's position on the equivalency of osteopathic medicine degrees from an accredited osteopathic medical school to medical degrees from an accredited medical school." The policy "recognizes a degree of Doctor of Osteopathic Medicine granted by an osteopathic medical school in the United States that was, at the time the degree was granted, accredited by the American Osteopathic Association as equivalent to a degree in medicine as defined in Clause (a) of Section 1 of *Ontario Regulation 865/93*."[86]

As for the other provinces and the territories, the national standard can be implemented once the respective governments pass enabling legislation that would allow their provincial colleges of physicians and surgeons and territorial health councils to formalize its adoption.

The new licensure standard was an initiative launched by the

Federation of Medical Regulatory Authorities of Canada (FRMRAC) and was partly a response to the national Agreement on Internal Trade (AIT), signed by the First Ministers Conference on the Economy on January 16, 2009. This standard had an important implication for doctors of osteopathic medicine; it enabled them to migrate with relative ease across borders within Canada.[87]

In Ontario, for example, the AIT became law in December 2009 with the passage of Bill 175, which requires the College to license applicants that hold a certificate in a Canadian jurisdiction if it is equivalent to a certificate issued by the College of Physicians and Surgeons of Ontario. If an equivalent out-of-province certificate is restricted, it permits the College to impose the same restrictions on the applicant's certificate in Ontario.

Some jurisdictions took action earlier than Ontario. In February 2009 Saskatchewan approved the protocols to the AIT. B.C. and Nova Scotia followed suit by passing legislation in October 2009.

Within a few years, however, teething problems cropped up. Provincial medical regulatory authorities faced the issue of "specially licensed physicians."

Restrictions on special licences, which can include "requiring the holders to be supervised by more experienced physicians and only allowing them to operate if the province has a shortage of the physicians' specialty, are not equivalent across provinces," a major daily paper reported on August 1, 2011, regarding the situation of Dr. Rubens Barbosa, an anaesthesiologist working in Edmundston, N.B., who had his application to transfer his licence to Ontario rejected.[88]

Dr. Yves Robert, then president of the Federation of Medical Regulatory Authorities of Canada and 2015 registrar of the Collège des médecins du Québec, responding to the debacle, told the newspaper reporter: "We are working on how we could facilitate for them a mobility from one jurisdiction to another taking into account the fact that they don't have a full licensure."[89]

The Canadian Osteopathic Association

In 2015, the Canadian Osteopathic Association (COA) turned 90. It was celebrated without fanfare by its osteopathic physician members who are estimated to be much fewer than 75 across Canada. However, its eight-person slate of officers headed by Joel Pash, a DO and anaesthesiologist registered with the Alberta College of Physicians and Surgeons, is continuing its reflection about where osteopathic medicine should be heading.

The stated goal of the COA is to "represent the osteopathic medical profession in all provincial and federal matters regarding legislation and licensure."[90]

Having worked long and hard over its 90-year history, the COA is likely pleased to be in the place where it is now—having gained recognition among the provincial and territorial medical authorities for the DO qualification.

The COA is, however, careful to distance practitioners who have a limited scope of practice utilizing only manual therapies.

The association has reminded the public on its website that a DO (osteopathic physician) has undertaken the same comprehensive medical education as a Canadian medical doctor as well as "comprehensive training in biomechanical assessment of the musculoskeletal system and treatment including osteopathic manipulative therapy."

"Following graduation from four years of intensive medical education," the group's website declares, "osteopathic physicians must further complete residency training in a specialty field of their choosing. They must then complete specialty certification examinations as well as medical licensure examinations required for registration with a provincial college of physicians and surgeons."

Historically, it took them multiple decades to get the medical authorities to recognize them as "doctors" with the title before their name provided they passed medical examinations set by Canada's two certifying medical institutions. That matter, however, is now metaphorically water under the bridge.

Today, a similar issue, in a different context, has raised its head again and this time it is not about the title "Doctor" and it does not have anything to do with the medical regulatory authorities. Instead, the COA is preoccupied with nomenclature: the use of the terms "osteopathy" or "osteopathic" by non-physician manual practitioners.

The COA's website describes the current situation: " . . . there are various practitioners presenting themselves as 'Osteopaths' or 'Osteopathic Practitioners', practising outside of legislation in Canada, who do not hold the comprehensive medical, surgical, and musculoskeletal training required for registration with a provincial medical authority in Canada."

Taking this message to a DO audience, two senior Canadian Osteopathic Association members (Dr. David Fiddler, of Ontario, and Dr. James Church, a Victoria, B.C.-based osteopathic physician who describes himself as a "third-generation" practitioner) stated the case to the mainly American readers of *The DO* magazine, published by the American Osteopathic Association: "We feel strongly that the use of osteopathic in titles of non-physicians in Canada is inappropriate. Such misuse is leading to considerable confusion in the public, government regulatory bodies and insurance companies, jeopardizing the integrity of the osteopathic medical profession while placing the public at risk."[91]

Drilling deeper into the controversy, Ted Findlay, DO, a former 16-year president of the COA, and a practising medical consultant and university faculty member in Calgary, had argued the group's case a year earlier, asking: "Is the practice of manual therapy without the capability to generate a complete diagnosis an appropriate use of the term "osteopathy"? Are our patients, especially those vulnerable during illness, sophisticated enough to differentiate between an osteopathic physician and an osteopathic practitioner?"[92]

What also vexed Findlay then and still does today is the non-physician practitioners who claim they practise "traditional osteopathy." "I believe this is a mistake with potentially dangerous implications for the profession," he once wrote.

A real definition of traditional osteopathy—if it exists at all—would be what doctors of osteopathy or osteopathic physicians do, he argued, pointing to the beginnings of osteopathy. "The administration of medications and surgery as well as obstetrics was practiced by the original founders of the profession, including Dr. Still, and they established hospitals for the appropriate provision of these aspects of care. In short, they were the most completely trained health-care providers in the world and used any tools available to help restore and enhance the health of patients."

The COA has indirectly blamed the Chicago-based Osteopathic International Alliance (OIA) for the situation. For example, the OIA admitted the Canadian Federation of Osteopaths (CFO), as an associate member, which represents provincial and territorial non-physician practitioners.

"It would appear that the Osteopathic International Alliance, which initially was established as a forum to discuss international osteopathic affairs, has become a haven for non-physician practitioners attempting to obtain international recognition and credibility regardless of training," stated the COA.

The COA's evidence has been that "there is now a movement by non-physician practitioners without any university qualifications and only a few weekends of "osteopathic" training to seek government recognition as "osteopathic practitioners." Despite these practitioners' minimal training (as little as 11 weekends), the Osteopathic International Alliance has accepted these groups into membership without any consideration of the negative impact on the osteopathic medical profession in Canada."[93]

Adding a supporting voice to the COA's position has been Santa Monica, CA–based Virginia M Johnson, DO, who has decried U.S. citizens going to Canada to study manual osteopathy. When they return to the United States, according to her, they hold themselves out as "DOs" as is the case with a physical therapist whom she cited "claim to have a 'certificate in osteopathy' from the Osteopathic College of Ontario (Canada)."

Dr. Johnson pointed to potential dangers. "Some of my patients come to me with untreated, progressing medical conditions—not to mention injuries sustained—after paying out of pocket to see such 'osteopaths,' unaware of the differences between these practitioners and DOs. The confusion and the danger to the public are the real issues," she wrote in a letter.[94]

When the COA was founded in 1925, it was recognized by the federal government as a national body representing osteopaths. It soon ran into financial problems causing it to go into hibernation. Seventeen years later, in 1942, it became active once again.

There is a dearth of information about what the COA had done since the years of the Second World War, but it has been just this past decade that some headway was made with regard to the "recognition of the DO diploma" issue.

Working closely with its American counterpart, the American Osteopathic Association, the COA has lobbied the Federation of Medical Regulatory Authorities of Canada (a national body that represents the 13 provincial and territorial medical regulatory authorities nationally and internationally), to ensure the American osteopathic medical degree is recognized under a pan-Canadian standard, called the "National Standard" for full and provisional licensure. Both these licences involve the physician practising as an MRP, or "most responsible physician."

"A national standard recognizes MD and DO as equivalent for registration in Canada. All provinces except Saskatchewan have made provisions for osteopathic physicians to register with their provincial college of physicians and surgeons or territorial health council. Saskatchewan plans to do so when it updates its *Health Professions Act*," said Findlay.

Another hurdle for the COA to overcome is that in early 2015 the Canadian National Standard did not recognize American board exams such as COMLEX-USA (Comprehensive Osteopathic Medical Licensing Examination) or the USMLE (United States Medical Licensing Examination).

According to Findlay, some provinces continue to recognize COMLEX and USMLE but they are not included within the requirements of the Canadian standard for inter-provincial portability.

"So if a graduate of an American osteopathic school wants to register with a college of physicians and surgeons, they may have to do, additionally, the MCC (Medical Council of Canada) exams as well as complete a residency," said Findlay.

The Canadian Osteopathic Medical Student Association, a group of medical student leaders dedicated to spreading knowledge of osteopathic medicine at home, provides assistance to current and potential U.S.-based Canadian students to "pursue their dream of practicing osteopathic medicine in Canada by helping (them) to navigate the requirements and processes," the group says on its website.[95]

The Canadian Federation of Osteopaths

She doesn't use the word "diplomacy" to describe her work but as president of the fledgling national body representing provincial and territorial manual osteopathic practitioners, Gail Abernethy is doing just that.

When she's not treating patients at her clinic in Sooke, B.C., the 43-year osteopathic practitioner and leader of the Canadian Federation of Osteopaths is steeped in carrying out the unenviable work of a diplomat.

Elected president in 2014 after serving as vice-president for four years, Abernethy is travelling on and off to foster relationships within Canada and around the world to resolve the issues facing Canadian manual osteopaths and to advance the interests of the profession that had its humble beginnings in 1981 with the opening of Canada's first manual osteopathic school in Quebec.

"There's a lot to keep on top of," said Abernethy. "There's a lot of different issues in the provinces and the territories as well as [those coming out of] the Osteopathic International Alliance and the European Federation of Osteopaths of which we are an associate member." Regarding these two international organizations, the CFO "must work together with them in this increasingly interconnected world," she declared.[96]

A key goal of the CFO is to collaborate with other Canadian health-care professions to increase the health-care delivery capacity for Canadians as well as to provide innovative solutions to the ever-increasing health-care challenges in the country.

Because provincial or territorial governments have yet to regulate the profession (although Quebec, since December 2014, launched a process to do so), an ongoing task of the CFO is to provide support to its members in their bid to secure regulatory status.

When the provinces and territories do decide in the coming years to follow Quebec's initiative, governments will be looking closely at the hallmarks of the profession that relate directly to public safety, such as education standards, codes of ethics and disciplinary measures employed by the groups that represent individual practitioners.

The CFO, an associate member of the Chicago-based Osteopathic International Alliance, upholds the 2010 World Health Organization training benchmarks that the alliance's members have all adopted, Abernethy said.

While the CFO has at least one organization representing Alberta, British Columbia, New Brunswick, Nova Scotia, Ontario and Quebec provinces—the territories are not yet members due to few or no known resident osteopathic manual practitioners—the national organization would welcome into its fold other groups from the provinces already represented, provided all their individual practitioners satisfy the minimum training guidelines set out in the WHO benchmarks. In 2013, "not all provinces have qualified, practicing osteopaths and professional associations," Gail Abernethy pointed out in a message on the OIA website.[97] Private institutions provide training for [manual] osteopaths in Canada and is typically a five-year, part-time, post-graduate professional training program for students who already have a previous health-care qualification, Abernethy added.

As the CFO, formed in 2007, moves ahead with its agenda to promote the profession as a whole, it inadvertently finds itself in an ideological clash with a kindred organization, the Canadian Osteopathic Association, the body that represents osteopathic physicians. These doctors are graduates of American Osteopathic Association-recognized osteopathic colleges in the United States and are also Licentiates of the Medical Council of Canada and have successfully completed a medical residency.

The COA has taken issue with Canadian osteopaths (who have varying titles—Osteopathic practitioner in British Columbia, Osteopathic Manual Therapist in Alberta, and Osteopathic Manual Practitioner in Ontario and Nova Scotia) on the latter's use of the terms "osteopathy" or "osteopathic" to describe their job title (see full details in the section of the Canadian Osteopathic Association elsewhere in this chapter).

The CFO's position is that the osteopathic physicians' organization "is not well informed," said Gail Abernethy, citing the position of international bodies such as the Osteopathic International Alliance and the World Health Organization that recognize osteopathic physicians and osteopaths as two professions with their separate modality or stream.

"It is important to note that not all osteopathic physicians are opposed to the idea of regulation and progress in the non-physician osteopath world. And the OIA has been a great help in the sense of providing a neutral forum where physician and non-physician osteopaths can discuss the issues they have in common," said Abernethy.

Speaking frankly, the CFO President Abernethy said, "We don't buy into their view of osteopathy and it's very important to know that very few people in the world buy into their view of osteopathy."

The OIA has 77 members which include the largest osteopathic organizations in the world, such as the German Association for Osteopathic Medicine, Osteopathy Australia, Fédération Suisse des Ostéopathes and the American Osteopathic Association that represents more than 80,000 osteopathic physicians. The COA is not a member of the OIA.

As for the near and distant future, "we'll just carry on communicating and trying to move forward with the profession as a whole with people who want to talk to us," said CFO President Abernethy.

Chapter 16—Osteopathy Today in Quebec and Ontario

A Bird's Eye View of Both Provinces

Douglas Ralph Fiddler and Jean-Guy Sicotte are both medical doctors but they also wear another health professional hat while making their rounds in hospital and private clinic settings.[98]

In addition to conventional medicine, they practise osteopathy. Hailing from Ontario and Quebec respectively, they are emblematic of a small core of health care professionals who are deeply engaged with two modalities of health care that have markedly different—like night and day—levels of official acceptance in Canada.

(Traditional medicine has been regulated for much more than a century in Canada whereas non-physician osteopathy is not regulated at all despite its widespread use by Canadians. Osteopaths have been seeking regulatory status since the 1980s while osteopathic physicians had been doing so since 1898 until they received some reprieve in the 2000s in the form of limited recognition in the provinces and territories.)

Dr. Fiddler, an emergency physician at the Haliburton Highlands Health Service in Minden, Ont., burned the midnight oil for several years in the U.S., graduating as a doctor of osteopathic medicine in the United States. But he had to demonstrate his mettle as a medical doctor in Ontario by having to pass several Canadian physician evaluation exams before he could practise medicine. Dr. Sicotte, on the other hand, had set his health professional sights first on family medicine, graduating in 1972 from the University of Montréal, and within two years felt the itch to take on osteopathy. He went to England and returned to Canada studying at both Sheffield University and Canada's and Montreal's first osteopathy school—Collège d'Études Ostéopathiques—and then re-established his practices in the Eastern Townships region of Quebec.

Whenever they put on their osteopathic hat, both doctors may apply non-invasive manual osteopathic treatments to patients; on the other hand, when they are practising as medical doctors they use the conventional tools of an MD such as drugs and surgery. If the patient agrees, they may use both therapeutic approaches for healing.

While the two straddle two widely different modalities in the healing arts, their representative institutions, such as the provincial colleges of physicians and surgeons, the Canadian Osteopathic Association, the Canadian Federation of Osteopaths and its provincial constituent members and Canada's second-tier government officials, find themselves in awkward conversations about the merits of each type of therapy and whether osteopathy should be sanctioned through regulation or whether osteopathic physicians really need to do Medical Council of Canada examinations and complete a residency.

As these sometimes heated discussions go on, those working in or aspiring to be in the front lines of either profession look on and wonder when it will all come to an end.

A breakthrough, however, lies in the horizon for osteopathy.

Observers predict that Quebec would likely be the first jurisdiction in Canada to create an "Ordre," or in the health professional lingo of English-speaking Canada, a regulatory college, to oversee osteopathy. The optimism stems from a December 17, 2014, invitation to the 1,200-osteopath strong Ostéopathique Québec, or the OQ and others, by the Office des professions du Québec, an advisory body to the government, to participate in a working group to recommend elements for a regulatory framework for the practice of osteopathy in the province.

As the two most populous provinces with more than 60 per cent of the country's 35 million population in 2014, Quebec and Ontario are the epicentres of Canada's osteopathic services industry.

It is estimated that the combined total of osteopathic manual practitioners (OMPs) and doctors of osteopathic medicine in both jurisdictions is 2,000 (with Quebec having more than 1,200 practitioners and Ontario with about 800 OMPs). Fewer than fifty osteopathic physicians practise in both jurisdictions, and all of them are in Ontario. In Ontario, the different licence classifications assigned to them are 'independent practice,' 'post-graduate education certificate,' and 'restricted certificate.'

In Quebec, in addition to the 1,200-osteopath member Ostéopathie Québec, there are a number of smaller advocacy associations of osteopaths. They include:

- The Corporation of Professional Osteopaths Quebec (Corporation des Professionnels en Ostéopathie du Québec, or CPOQ);
- Collège des Ostéopathes Canadiens (COC);

- Canadian Society for Traditional Osteopathy (So.Ca.T.O.);
- Syndicat Professionnel des Ostéopathes du Québec (SPOQ);
- L'Association québecoise des ostéopathes (AQO);
- Association RITMA;
- Canadian Union of Professional Osteopaths (CUPO);
- La Société des Ostéopathes du Québec (SOQ) also known as L'Ordre des Ostéopathes du Québec; and
- L'Association Canadienne des thérapeutes en Médecines Douces (ACTMD).

In Ontario, the Ontario Association of Osteopathic Manual Practitioners (OAO) is one of the larger non-profit professional associations of osteopathic manual practitioners—with 260 active members in January 2015.[99] Other Ontario groups that advocate for the profession include:

- Osteopathic and Alternative Medicine Association (OOAMA);
- Ontario Association of Osteopathy and Natural Medicine (OAONM);
- Ontario Osteopathic Association (OOA);
- Ontario College of Osteopathic Rehabilitation Sciences (OCORS);
- Ontario Council of Drugless Osteopathy (OCDO); and
- International Osteopathic Association (IOA).

In both provinces, there are close to two dozens of osteopathy schools that have been established since the first one—the Collège d'Études Ostéopathique—opened its doors in Montreal in 1981.

In Quebec, other schools include:

- Education Institute of Osteopathy Quebec;
- l'Institut de l'enseignement de l'ostéopathie du Québec (IEOQ);
- L'Académie d'ostéopathie de Montréal (AOM);
- Quebec Sutherland Osteopathy Academy (Académie Sutherland d'Ostéopathie du Québec (ASOQ);
- Collège D'Ostéopathie du Québec à Québec (COQQ);
- Le Collège Canadien de la Médecine Ostéopathique (CCMO); and
- Collège D'Ostéopathie du Québec à Montréal (COQM).

In Ontario, more than half a dozen manual osteopathy schools dot the southern part of the province. They include:

- Canadian Academy of Osteopathy (CAO);
- Canadian College of Osteopathy (CCO);
- National Academy of Osteopathy (NAO);
- Ontario School of Osteopathy and Alternative Medicine (OSO);
- The Osteopathic College of Ontario (OCO);
- Southern Ontario College of Osteopathy (SOCO); and
- London College of Osteopathy (LSO)

Most are located in the Greater Toronto Area (GTA) that comprises the City of Toronto and the four regional municipalities surrounding it—Durham, Halton, Peel, and York. The London College of Osteopathy is located in the City of London.

Quebec

Osteopaths

In the eyes of Quebec politicians and public health analysts, the province has the potential to become the first regulated Canadian jurisdiction for osteopathy by virtue of its large, growing professional osteopath population as well as Quebecers' dedicated use of osteopathic manual therapy.

A Fraser Institute researcher discovered that while Canadians' use of osteopathy doubled between 1997 and 2006, much of this occurred in Quebec, where use increased to 11 per cent from 3 per cent during this period. In addition, the number of Quebecers having "total/a lot of confidence" in osteopathy was 89 per cent, the highest among twenty-two alternative therapies with chiropractic care coming in at 81 per cent, Nadeem Esmail, former head of health system performance studies at the Fraser Institute, wrote in his 2007 report on complementary and alternative medicine.[100]

It was perhaps no big surprise to the board of directors and members of the Ostéopathique Québec, the province's largest, and therefore the most credible osteopath group, when the Office des professions du Québec, the government's health advisory body, launched a new consultation process on December 17, 2014, to research the possibilities of including manual osteopathy as a part of Quebec's current professions system which comprises fifty-three regulated professions.

(According to the Conseil interprofessionel du Québec {Quebec Inter-professional Council}, the province's professions system comprises "various institutions which, based on their jurisdictions and responsibilities, play a role in overseeing Quebéc's fifty-three regulated professions and developing and promoting the mission to protect the public.")[101]

The pre-2014 Christmas Day communiqué established ". . . a working group to follow the recommendations of the [work] of two previous committees and to recommend the creation of a distinct Ordre which will have the responsibility to regulate the practice [of osteopathy]."[102] The tasks ahead for the working group will probably include consulting with Quebec's osteopathy schools and the province's professional associations of osteopaths.

The Office des professions du Québec's reference to "two previous committees" concerns a "comité d'expert" set up in 2008 that prepared a report in 2011.[103] According to a former president of the Canadian Federation of Osteopaths that took part in the comité d'expert deliberations, some osteopath participants were chosen because they had previous experience in allied health care fields, such as nursing, massage therapy, athletic rehabilitation therapy, and acupuncture before osteopath training.[104]

In a few years beyond 2015, observers believe Quebec may pass a law regulating osteopathy. This would realize the quintessential dream of all non-physician osteopaths and should that occur, Quebec would become a trailblazer for the profession in Canada.

Events Prior to Dec. 17, 2014 Quebec Announcement

The seeds of change were sown in the mid-1980s.

When the first cohort of graduates of the Collège d'Études Ostéopathiques, the first manual osteopathic training institution in Quebec and in Canada, they realized the significance of organizing as a group for interfacing with future governments for regulatory purposes.

Under the leadership of medical doctor Roger Robitaille, DO, and Thérèse Menard, DO, a voluntary association of osteopaths called the Le Régistre des Ostéopathes du Québec (ROQ) was formed to help prepare the students to practise under self-regulation. The ROQ was set up as a cooperative with the students being its "members" and having a direct say in how the co-op developed.

The students also created the L'Association des Ostéopathes du

Québec (ADOQ) with Robitaille and Menard also at the helm. The registry "was the base for a future corporation or professional order, for the protection of the people." Both these interest groups profess to have the same rules of deontology (that is, the ethics around duty, and moral obligation) and "to control the professional behaviour" of members.[105]

The founders of the ADOQ had another objective in mind for this organization: it was to manage the administrative issues in establishing the profession, such as securing malpractice insurance, and developing arrangements with insurance companies for the reimbursement of treatments in extended health policies.

In 2012, a merger of the ROQ and the ADOQ resulted in the creation of Ostéopathie Québec (OQ), with more than 1,200 members. The OQ, in 2015, is the single largest group of manual osteopaths in Canada.

Soon after the mid-2000s, as the two groups' membership grew, their leaders began strategizing about obtaining regulatory status for manual osteopathy. They began lobbying the Office des professions du Québec, members of the National Assembly and public policy managers in the health and education ministries.

Two smaller groups had also been adding their voices to the chorus for statutory recognition. The Corporation of Professional Osteopaths Québec (CPOQ) and Collège des Ostéopathes Canadiens (COC). The COC has described itself as "the first association of osteopaths in Quebec dedicated exclusively to healthcare professionals" and provides services for both representation as a group to the government as well as to "teach osteopathy and provide [continuing] education to its members. We then developed a code of conduct that incorporates the basic elements of the chiropractors and doctors, and an internal regulation that defines a code of conduct," the COC wrote on its website.[106]

Osteopath Training

La belle province has the distinction of being the first province in Canada to introduce manual osteopathy. It all started through an entrepreneurial educational project by Philippe Druelle, DO, and Dr. Jean-Guy Sicotte. They founded Canada's first traditional osteopathy school, the Collège d'Études Ostéopathiques de Montreal (the Montreal College of Osteotherapy) on March 11, 1981.[107]

Druelle, then a recent immigrant from France, had recognized the potential for manual osteopathy to help alleviate suffering among the public in a country where medical authorities have historically ignored the major regulatory concerns of doctors of osteopathic medicine. A complementary school called the Centre Ostéopathique du Québec (COQ) was established four years later.

Institut d'enseignement de l'ostéopathie du Québec

The offering by the Institut d'enseignement de l'ostéopathie du Québec in Montreal is a three-year training program with two classes per week and other options. "Following the first session, students enrolled in the educational osteopathy Institute of Québec can start his own osteopathic practice identifying himself as a student of osteopathy [at] the academic Institute of Québec, have liability insurance malpractice, be reimbursed fees. At the end of his training, the student will have gained experience . . . ," the school's website says.[108]

L'Académie d'ostéopathie de Montréal

The course outline at the L'Académie d'ostéopathie de Montréal (AOM) is based on the 2010 training benchmarks developed by the World Health Organization. "The high standards mean that graduates of AOM who have completed this program will be able to practice [osteopathy] in all Canadian provinces," the AOM said on its website.[109]

In revising its course syllabus, the Académie D'Ostéopathie de Montréal collaborated with a health research group at L'Université du Québec à Montréal. The outcome is a "repository of professional competence [guidelines] required for future osteopathic graduates of its establishment."

To strengthen its offerings, the AOM partnered with the Université du Québec à Trois-Rivières (UQTR) to improve its course in dissection. Not one to overlook the importance of social media, the AOM has been the first osteopathy school to use the Internet to broadcast lessons to the students working away from the classroom.[110]

Académie Sutherland d'Ostéopathie du Québec

Guy Voyer started the Académie Sutherland d'Ostéopathie du Québec in 2000. The school's objective is to develop its osteopathic students so they are able "to choose among [a] panoply of tools at the right moment. Under no circumstances do we want our students to become technicians repeating osteopathic techniques."[111]

The school stresses the importance of personal individual study of the content of the theoretical content prior to each course, to make it possible for teachers to focus on the practical work.[112]

Graduates of the six-year part-time course receive an osteopathic diploma (DO) and an International Osteopathic Diploma (IDO) issued by the Federal European Register of Osteopaths.

College d'Ostéopathie du Québec á Montréal

The College d'Ostéopathie du Québec à Montréal (COQM) or the Quebec College of Osteopathy in Montreal, awards a DO degree when students complete bachelor of science of osteopathy courses as well as pass the practical, theoretical, and oral final examinations at the passing grade of 60 per cent.[113] It also offers training leading to a Ph.D. in osteopathy (Ph.D. DO).

École professionnelle des ostéopathes du Québec

A major focus in the osteopathy training at École professionnelle des ostéopathes du Québec (EPOQ), or the Professional School of Osteopaths of Quebec, is developing students' case management skills to effectively meet their clients' health needs through communication and the proper use of resources. Starting in September 2014, it instituted a new curriculum with more than 1,000 hours of clinical training.[114]

Other Schools in Quebec

There is no substantive information available regarding these organizations: Le Collège Canadien de la Médecine Ostéopathique (CCMO), also called the Canadian College of Osteopathic Medicine; Collège d'Ostéopathie Supérieur du Québec; and Collège D'Etiopathie Supérieur du Québec (CESQ).

Osteopathic Physicians

The Collège des médecins du Québec, the medical regulatory body for the province, recognizes the diploma of doctor of osteopathy (DO) awarded by U.S. colleges of osteopathic medicine. The schools, however, must be accredited by the Commission on Osteopathic College Accreditation of the American Osteopathic Association on the date the diploma is granted.[115]

As in other provinces, to obtain a medical practice permit, they must be Licentiates of the Medical Council of Canada and successfully complete a residency with either the Royal College of Physicians and Surgeons of Canada or the College of Family Physicians of Canada.

The current limited recognition of the status of DOs came about after their historically long lobbying effort aimed at the Collège des médecins du Québec and the provincial government and following presentations by both the Canadian Osteopathic Association and the American Osteopathic Association.

The COA and AOA had reached out, as early as 1981, to the Federation of Medical Regulatory Authorities of Canada (FMRAC) on this issue. The national body has since developed a "National Standard" for all medical doctors, and now osteopathic medical doctors, to meet before they can be fully licensed to practise. And, in June 2013, the Quebec medical regulator signed an agreement in principle with their peer regulators of the other provinces and the territories to introduce it.

(FMRAC is a national organization representing the 13 provincial and territorial medical regulatory authorities.)

In 1928 and 1935 the Collège des médecins du Québec, responding to complaints from the medical doctors, brought charges against thirteen DOs alleging they were illegally practising medicine, but later dropped them after a negotiated settlement. In exchange, the DOs withdrew a bill that was making its way through the Quebec parliament. They also had to agree that an MD degree was required by them to be considered for licensure.

In its bid to carry out its mandate, the medical regulatory body has been vigilant about monitoring osteopathic manual practitioners practising "medicine" as defined in the province's medical laws. "The medical establishment therefore keeps a close eye on practitioners who may try to tell their clients they're just as qualified as doctors to treat them," a CTV Montreal journalist reported in 2014 when manual osteopath and naturopath Ken Montizambert faced twelve charges of illegally practising medicine, including writing prescriptions. The initial allegations were made by the Collège des médecins du Québec. The courts handed down an injunction on July 21 in the same year restricting his scope of practice.[116]

Ostéopathie Québec (OQ), the largest provincial association of osteopaths, did not defend Montizambert's actions. The OQ's president in 2014, Isabelle Coindre, told the media, "This is the type of the problem that shows we need a regulation for osteopathy in Quebec."[117] The sixty-three-year old osteopathic manual practitioner, who runs Tri-Med Clinic in Pointe Claire, vowed to appeal the court decision.

Ontario

Osteopathic Physicians

For osteopathic physicians who graduated from osteopathy schools in the United States, the die was cast not too long ago.

At its 80 College St. headquarters in Toronto one evening in September 2003, the governing body of the College of Physicians and Surgeons of Ontario (CPSO) adopted a policy to recognize "a degree of Doctor of Osteopathic Medicine granted by an osteopathic medical school in the United States that was, at the time the degree was granted, accredited by the American Osteopathic Association as equivalent to a degree in medicine."[118] For those U.S. graduates, the news about the new policy became a game-changer in their professional lives and one they had anticipated since the provincial government passed *Ontario Regulation 865/93*, under the *Medicine Act*, 1991 a decade earlier. Clause (a) of section 1 of that law had set out the standards and qualifications for a certificate of registration that the CSPO issues to medical graduates to allow an independent practice.

It may be hard, for some, to contemplate that slightly fewer than a hundred years before, the traditional medical community vilified osteopathy as something short of evil. It was commonplace to read accounts in Toronto newspapers reporting that leaders of the medical profession had allegedly referred to osteopathy as "a cult" and expressed other non-flattering statements about the profession (for more details on Ontario's osteopathic physicians and their interactions with the government and the conventional medical community, please see the Ontario section of the chapter in this book, titled "Thinking Hands in Canada Through the Decades").

Osteopaths (called Osteopathic Manual Practitioners in Ontario)

Since the humble beginnings of traditional osteopathy in the 1980s in Quebec, the profession has matured while becoming a viable and popular health-care service in the province, with estimated patient visits in the range of hundreds of thousands in the immediate past few years.

Alongside other natural medical practices such as acupuncture, traditional Chinese medicine, naturopathy, and massage therapy, osteopathy holds its own but is unregulated. Despite its appeal to Ontario's increasingly health-conscious residents who now also demand and buy aplenty non-GMO, gluten-free natural health products (food supplements like vitamins, minerals, fruit pectin) and organically grown fruits and vegetables, it is not a health-care service that can be easily accessible.

As a partly subsidized item available at one time years ago through OHIP, the Ontario Health Insurance Plan, it came under scrutiny by cost-cutting politicians and became delisted after health budget reviews. So it remains largely affordable to middle class families and others.

Services from osteopathic practitioners are not cheap. The cost of a one-hour treatment with an osteopathic manual practitioner, for example, range from $100 to $150 per visit. So should members of the public desire it to be part of their health regime, they must be willing to reach into their pocketbook.

Even those with liberal extended health insurance plans that cover osteopathic treatments,. often find they have to fork out quite a bit from their wallets, as coverage only goes so far. In some plans, such as Great West Life's, the benefit amount is limited to a maximum for an osteopath recognized by the insurance company, of $300 per insured person per calendar year (Basic and Comprehensive Plans) and $400 per insured person per calendar year (Premier Plan)[119]

Looking for Osteopathic Health Care: Ontario Consumers' Two Choices

Ontario consumers seeking osteopathic health-care services can choose two types of this non-invasive manual medicine. The first kind is traditional osteopathy, also known as classical osteopathy, osteopathic manual therapy, non-physician osteopathy, osteopathic manual manipulation, or osteopathic manual medicine. The second type is the same as the first but can be administered by osteopathic physicians (in Ontario, these physicians practise conventional medicine and may use traditional osteopathy as a complement to what they practise.). Most osteopathic manual practitioners are graduates of osteopathy schools that operate across Canada. Many have learned osteopathy from overseas bodies like the British School of Osteopathy in England, and generally hold a DOMP (or DO(MPT) in England) designation or their equivalents such as a BSc Hons. in osteopathy, Bachelor of Osteopathy (BOst) or BOstMed, or a masters degree (MOst) or a master in osteopathic manipulative sciences or M.OMSC.

For instance, Heidi Van Vliet, a registered massage therapist for more than ten years, crossed over to osteopathic practice after receiving the M.OMSC in 2012 from the Canadian Academy of Osteopathy. She runs Osteopathically You in Alliston, Ontario, a community within the Town of New Tecumseh in central Ontario. At the Lifetime Wellness Center in Windsor, Andrea Balkwill, an osteopathic manual practitioner in an eight-person professional care team, graduated from the three-year osteopathy program at Mississauga's Southern Ontario College of Osteopathy following obtaining a bachelor of human kinetics degree from the University of Windsor.

The other stream in osteopathy is osteopathic medicine that is provided by doctors of osteopathic medicine, also officially called, in Ontario, osteopaths or osteopathic physicians. They hold a DO degree from accredited U.S. osteopathic colleges and also always hold a licence, issued by the College of Physicians and Surgeons of Ontario. In addition to their skill sets in manipulation medicine—the substance of what osteopathic manual practitioners do—they have certified knowledge and experience in conventional medicine.

For instance, in Newmarket, Ontario, Amy H. Wong, MD, graduated as a doctor of osteopathic medicine from the NYIT College of Osteopathic Medicine in New York in 2002. She also completed a U.S. residency recognized by both the American Osteopathic Association and the Accreditation Council for Graduate Medical Education. The residency included licensing examinations on osteopathic medical knowledge and clinical skills considered essential for osteopathic generalist physicians to practise medicine without supervision.

After she returned to Ontario, she became a family medicine specialist after passing the certification examinations of the College of Family Physicians of Canada and the American Board of Family Medicine.

Counting the Numbers

The treatment rooms of hundreds of Ontario-based osteopathic manual practitioners are sprinkled across the complementary health care services provider landscape from Sarnia to Ottawa and from Thunder Bay to Kingston.

In Canada's most populous province, with 13.5 million residents in 2013,.there is one osteopathic physician for approximately every 500,000 residents.

(South of the border, a much brighter global osteopathic medicine picture exists. In the United States with a population of 315 million in 2013,.there were more than 82,000 osteopathic physicians practising or one osteopathic physician available for approximately 3,800 Americans.)

On the other hand, the number of osteopathic manual practitioners stands at over 800 and is swelling with each passing year as graduates of the half-dozen or so manual osteopathic schools in Canada enter the market. The 2014 estimate of 800 is based on the listings of members (some groups' membership listings were inaccessible) on the website of eight Ontario associations representing the practitioners. The groups are:

- Ontario Association of Osteopathic Manual Practitioners (OAO);
- Ontario Federation of Osteopathic Professionals (OFOP);
- Ontario Osteopathic Association (OOA);
- Ontario Osteopathic and Alternative Medicine Association (OOAMA);
- Ontario Association of Osteopathy and Natural Medicine (OAONM);
- Ontario Council of Drugless Osteopathy (OCDO);
  Ontario College of Osteopathic Rehabilitation Sciences (OCORS);
- Ontario Council of Drugless Osteopathy (OCDO); and
- International Osteopathic Association (IOA).

In August 2014, according to the College of Physicians and Surgeons of Ontario, there were forty-three osteopathic medical doctors on its registry. Members are issued various categories or "classes" of certificates of registration, and each class specifies an authorized type of practice.[120]

Of that number, seventeen held what the college deems a "Certificate of Registration authorizing Postgraduate Education" which means they can get into a supervised practice after graduation from medical school, and were attending postgraduate (residency) training at an Ontario medical school. This practice opportunity is one of the school's requirements. They are allowed to prescribe drugs for in-patients or outpatients of a clinical teaching unit at the school, and patients get free medical services.

Seven doctors of osteopathic medicine were issued a "Certificate of Registration authorizing Independent Practice."This permitted them to undertake an independent practice in the areas of medicine in which they were educated and experienced.

Nineteen held restricted certificates, which meant they had to practice under specific terms and conditions described on the certificate.

Meeting Challenges

As providers of what is essentially a non-publicly funded health care service, osteopathic manual practitioners have learned to find creative ways to make a living. According to Pay Scale Human Capital salary calculator, the median compensation for an osteopath is $93,599 (based on National Salary data based on 50 per cent of those who provided information for the December 10, 2014 report).

Their kindred practitioners, osteopathic physicians who are licensed for an independent practice as they are paid through the Ontario Health Insurance Plan, are better off: $115,732 per year as the median salary (with 153 respondents reporting for the December 10, 2014 survey.[121]

In metropolitan areas such as Kitchener-Cambridge-Waterloo, Ottawa-Gatineau, and the Greater Toronto Area, the high cost of managing a business has pushed budget-conscious practitioners to partner with like-minded natural health practitioners to reduce operating expenses by sharing space and offering a bundle of under-one-roof multi-disciplinary services.

In those sprawling metropolises, consumers welcome this kind of one-stop "shopping" to avoid driving across a city multiple times to get natural health consultations.

One good early example in Ontario of this inter-professional collaboration in delivering health care took place in Toronto in 2002 when osteopathic manual practitioners worked side by side with eight established primary care medical professionals at the Artists' Health Centre, run by the Artists' Health Centre Foundation, at the Toronto General Hospital.

Since then, this collaborative sharing-practice-space model has been replicated dozens of times.

In Burlington, C. Gus Kandilas, Doug Mathieu and Darren Wharrie are three osteopathic practitioners who form part of a health care team at the Burlington Centre for Osteopathic and Athletic Therapy that opened its doors in 2007. The clinic also includes two registered massage therapists and a traditional Chinese medicine-acupuncture specialist. Fifty kilometers away north, in Guelph, Balance Integrated Health Solutions, offers this south-western Ontario city of over 120,000 residents, a roster of nine registered massage therapists, two osteopathic practitioners who double up as yoga instructors, and a naturopathic doctor.

In Toronto's posh downtown Village of Yorkville and one of Canada's most exclusive shopping destinations, Satori Health & Wellness is a giant in the complementary health care industry: it has twenty-five practitioners on its payroll that includes four osteopathic manual practitioners, specialists in acupuncture, traditional Chinese medicine, orthotics, chiropractic, naturopathy, and registered massage therapy offering four kinds of massages, including pre-natal.

The mushrooming of such private natural health care centres that has opened the door to new practising opportunities for manual osteopathic practitioners has been largely pushed by demand from a growing natural health-oriented public for alternate and complementary health services.

Markham, Ont. – based Iva Lloyd, known in the naturopathic professional community for her history book on Canadian naturopathic medicine, wrote in 2009 that "[a]lthough conventional medicine still holds the monopoly on health care, there is a growing acceptance and understanding of alternative medicine. The scientific model is still the overriding of focus of conventional medicine, yet the holistic and natural therapeutic methods are being recognized as an integral part of disease prevention and health promotion."[122]

In 2015, without the professional mantle of being formally regulated in legislation, osteopathic manual practitioners have yet to be invited to join the inner circle of conventional medicine. Having regulatory status, they have a great chance to be invited to join inter-professional teams such as Family Health Teams and Nurse Practitioner-Led Clinics and work in hospitals to help triage patients with musculoskeletal issues.

How Health Trends Influenced Osteopathy

The current high point in public demand in the 21st century for osteopathy is, interestingly, a repeat of an earlier historical period in Ontario when osteopathic services, delivered by doctors of osteopathic medicine, manual osteopaths' predecessors, had a heyday last century.

Tracey L. Adams, sociology chair at the University of Western Ontario who did extensive research in 2012 on osteopathy's pioneers in Ontario described the osteopathy scene last century:

In the early 1920s, osteopathic physicians in Ontario had every reason to feel optimistic about the future of their profession in the province. American-trained osteopaths had practised in Ontario since the turn of the twentieth century, and the profession appeared to be coming into its own. Osteopaths' patient base was strong and growing, and they had achieved a general level of acceptance, especially in urban areas.[123]

Several decades earlier, health journalist Charlotte Gray, a contributing editor to the *Canadian Medical Association Journal*, described how that consumer trend gathered steam. Writing in that magazine in 1999, she noted there have been ". . . changing expectations outside [conventional] medicine's institutional walls. Canadians are increasingly distrustful of "scientific" medicine and eager to investigate therapies drawn from sources as varied as Chinese medicine and homeopathy."[124]

Acknowledging this shift in public attitudes, the powerful medical regulator, the College of Physicians and Surgeons of Ontario, had earlier chimed in with policy No. 3-11, enacted in 1997 and updated twice by its Council, the college's decision-making body. The policy's introduction states: "In increasing numbers, patients are looking to complementary medicine for answers to complex medical problems, strategies for improved wellness or relief from acute medical symptoms."[125]

The osteopathic services industry—and those in dozens of other natural therapies—certainly has benefited from the medical regulator's acknowledgement of public demand for complementary health. Currently, osteopathic manual and other natural therapy practitioners are enjoying a boom in business. This newly found prosperity has plenty to do with changing demographics. The aging baby boomers—those born between 1946 and 1965—combined with a long growing disenchantment among a growing portion of the public with the promises of conventional medicine are pushing the demand for osteopathic and allied natural medicine services.

Observes Dundas Bradley, an osteopathic manual practitioner who runs THINK Osteopathy clinic in London: "I am getting more and more patients who are just fed up with the medical system and as the population grows older, that demographic [consisting] of the baby boomers wants more and more non-medical interventions for their pain and other problems."[126]

Orleans-based osteopathic manual practitioner and physiotherapist Chantal Roy whose main clientele lives in suburban Ottawa and is mainly in the 40-70 age group agrees. "As people retire they want to stay healthy, they will want to consult [with us] more. I think they lost faith in medical doctors."[127]

"They [medical doctors] don't have much to offer sometimes and clients say they would go to the doctors and get painkillers [but] they would like [them] to treat the cause," she added. "They want to stay healthy longer after sixty-five and still be active and travel—they are more conscious about their health and they want to take the means to get better." Osteopathic services are one of the means, Roy noted.

Osteopathic Culture

To read what Toronto osteopathic manual practitioner Miyako Kurihashi says about her job is to be reminded of the values embodied in the philosophy of Osteopathy's founder, Dr. Andrew Taylor Still who once wrote: "Osteopathy is to me a very sacred science. It is sacred because it is a healing power through all nature."[128]

Kurihashi, a ten-year osteopath at Toronto's Satori Health & Wellness clinic, has expressed the hope that "all osteopath manual practitioners [in Canada would] be learning and evolving under the laws of osteopathic principles and nature's law. All should be practised with the intention of sincere heart, [and] pure love," she wrote in an e-mail.[129]

In Mississauga, Michael Todosijevic, a graduate of the Canadian College of Osteopathy, talks about "a culture of care" – that is firmly in place at his Osteopathic Therapy Centre in Mississauga.[130]

For Ottawa-based Angela Wangda, both a physiotherapist and manual osteopath, osteopathy's key value is to practise along "a total mind-body-spirit continuum." This means to a great extent she feels a strong responsibility to those needing her help—her patients whose ages range from 40 to 103—for a return to a state of balance and harmony.

By using science-based approaches with a strong grounding in physiology and anatomy and the "research we have, we will be better at that so we can justify, on a physiological level, what we're doing" to deliver good care to patients,"[131]

Says twenty-year practitioner Janet Walker, of Toronto Osteopathy, "I combine strong intuitive skills, an inquisitive nature, and a thorough understanding of health sciences."[132]

Part of the mission of the two-practitioner team of Nancy Medeiros and Jared Postance, who operate two clinics called Paths 2 Vitality in Toronto, along with a naturopathic doctor, is to "unite mind, body and spirit . . . in every way possible." Both declare they "recognize that the human body is a self-regulating and self-healing entity and will strive for health naturally when given the appropriate guidance," adding that they "believe in a well-rounded, evidence-based holistic approach rooted in science.".[133]

The common theme underlying the expressions of these osteopathic manual practitioners is their identification with the values embedded in the traditional or classical principles of osteopathy's founder, Dr. Andrew Taylor Still. They get their sense of validation not just from getting their DOMP, or diploma in osteopathic manual therapy, but aligning their thinking and daily practice with an osteopathic medical philosophy.

In the authors' survey of Ontario's osteopathic manual practitioners, the dominant narrative is that they see themselves as professionals with practices at which they can use their classical manual manipulation skills based on the focus of the profession's founder on the power of self-healing as well as provide sensitive client care and to do so based on current and new evidence-based research that may be available.

Those contacted give possible credence to the osteopathic textbooks that claim they "treat people, not conditions."

The Making of an Osteopath in Ontario

For more than twenty years William R. Fitzsimmons has been the chief student head-hunter for the most prestigious post-secondary educational institution in the world. His job at Harvard University is to identify and approve, using what he calls a "holistic admissions" model, those applicants who are most worthy to populate Harvard's classrooms. For him, as admissions and financial aid dean, and his team, for example, the 2014 "search for the Class of 2017 was based not just on test scores, but on the activities, adversities, and other measures that reveal an applicant's character, achievements, and talents."[134]

The purpose of tough entry requirements is, according to education experts, to find the right students with the best potential for development and to help assure the larger society is served through their contributions after they get out of school.

With osteopathic manual training, the goal is that the right students would be transformed into highly competent practitioners by graduation day and will have a telling impact on their patients by eliminating their pains and also providing lifestyle counselling as a preventive measure.

But observers of the health care scene are raising issues about entry standards for entering the health professions and the effectiveness of the education they are getting. Because manual osteopathy is unregulated in Ontario, but osteopathic medicine is, the province's manual osteopathy schools have varying standards about whom they will admit as students.

This situation does not deter observers from raising contentious questions such as:

- How good or great are Ontario's osteopathic educational organizations in the absence of government regulation?
- How good or great are these schools in preparing students in an environment with changing health care expectations?
- How good or great are the clinical training guidelines and algorithms for manual osteopathy and the new possible approaches to improve their effectiveness?
- How good or great are the schools in helping their charges deal with the needs of an aging population or working in a team-based environment.[135]

Training the Students

The more than half-a-dozen manual osteopathic training organizations are private career colleges and stand outside of the province's publicly funded network of twenty universities, twenty-four community colleges and a skilled trades management system.

Since manual osteopathy is viewed by both the federal Department of Employment and Social Development and Statistics Canada as a professional occupation in health diagnosing and treating. Manual osteopathy comes under the NOC (National Occupational Classification) code number 3123 which describes what people in that field do, and the schools of osteopathy do not require approval from the Superintendent of Private Career Colleges at Ontario's ministry of training, colleges and universities, to operate.

According to Gail Abernethy, the vice-president of the Canadian Federation of Osteopaths in 2013, training at private career colleges is typically a five-year, part time, post graduate training for students who already have a previous health care qualification. Full time programs are becoming more available.[136]

The federated body of manual osteopaths only allows provincial and territorial manual osteopathic associations into its membership roster that meet or exceed WHO (World Health Organization) benchmarks of education as detailed by the world body's *Benchmarks for Training in Osteopathy*.

The benchmark system establishes a worldwide standard for the qualification, accreditation or licensing of practitioners of osteopathy, and according to the WHO, should support integration of manual osteopathy into the national health care system.

Ontario Schools of Osteopathy

Six Ontario schools—the Canadian College of Osteopathy, National Academy of Osteopathy, the Ontario School of Osteopathy and Alternative Medicine, Southern Ontario College of Osteopathy, the Osteopathic College of Ontario and the London College of Osteopathy— are briefly described here:[137]

Canadian College of Osteopathy

Students at the Toronto campus of the Canadian College of Osteopathy graduate with the trade-marked designation, DOMP. This is awarded after they completing five years of study of "traditional osteopathy" and one to two years of independent philosophical, clinical or experimental research. They also obtain the D.Sc.O. designation that indicates completion of a thesis.

The diploma program consists of 2100 hours of class time that has a particular focus that includes theory and the methodology, practical and clinical elements related to it. According to its website, students also study and practise the "techniques from the four disciplines, osteo-articular, cranial-sacral, visceral normalization and fascial release."[138]

Osteopathic manual trainees at CCO are required to do a mandatory review course three times during their program. "This exercise provides an excellent review of the previous year's material, allows the students to take the first steps towards conducting research, and permits each student to become informed and proficient in a selected area of osteopathy," its website notes.

In a wide-ranging interview, school Principal Brad McCutcheon said while the school's curriculum will always strictly adhere to the classical principles and philosophy of osteopathy taught by the founder of osteopathy, the late Dr. Andrew T. Still, the school might consider incorporating in its future training "new ways of applying" recent advancements in neurophysiology.

"Advanced research in neurophysiology has over the last five to ten years led to a collection of discoveries," he said. "Different types of neuro-transmitters and receptors we were previously unaware of in the spinal cord have come to light. These receptors can be affected by certain types of pharmaceuticals."

According to McCutcheon, it may be possible to later adapt this knowledge into the college's medical science courses and develop new techniques that students can learn to improve the interactions of these receptors. This could ultimately translate into better treatments for future patients.

Asked whether osteopathy's pioneers would get upset by introducing newfangled technologies, McCutcheon said "Dr. Still always did a lot of D.O., that is 'dig on', which means, it stands for us to learn more every day and not get stuck in old routines. So using that quote only, I can say that he would be pretty excited."

The school principal also said graduates can apply, as a top-up, for entry into a B.Sc. (Hons.) Osteopathy program offered by the British College of Osteopathic Medicine in England. "Right now it's just a way a graduate can upgrade to, if they want, from a diploma to a degree," he said. The curriculum for the ten-month honours degree, which is officially referred to in the British Isles as "the BSc (Hons) Osteopathy Conversion Degree for Diplomates," is monitored by the British College of Osteopathic Medicine, a specialist osteopathic educational institution in London, England.

The Toronto CCO belongs to a network of several osteopathy training institutions across Canada, including Halifax, Montreal, Vancouver and Winnipeg. According to the CCO website, the group, called the Association of Traditional Osteopathic Colleges of Canada, was established to ensure their educational program has "uniform standards of curriculum, teaching and evaluation" with supervision from its Academic Council that supervises its examinations, protocols and thesis submissions, and presentations.

National Academy of Osteopathy

The National Academy of Osteopathy (NAO) in Toronto awards a diploma in osteopathic manual practice for full-time students who complete one year of studies. Those students would not have had prior health education. At the same time, it awards the same qualification to students who have prior health education, such as registered massage therapists and nurses, and passed its examinations after six months of full-time study. The NAO also offers a fellowship program in osteopathic rehabilitation sciences and programs to certify persons applying for jobs as assistants in osteopathic offices, or in osteopathic manipulative or auxiliary osteopathy therapies.

The NAO says on its website that its graduates are eligible to receive two years of advanced credit in order to complete the DO (Doctor of Osteopathy) program at the National University of Medical Sciences

(NUMSS) in Spain. The college adds that those with a degree in the health and medical sciences can receive three years of advanced credit and are eligible to complete the DO program in one year as a full time student.

The National University of Medical Sciences offers Category 3 (one year full-time), Category 2 (two years' full-time), Category 1 (four years' full-time) programs leading to the degree, as well as a Bachelor of Science in osteopathy.[139]

(According to a policy adopted by the Council of the College of Physicians and Surgeons of Ontario, only DO degrees awarded by accredited osteopathic colleges in the United States are recognized in Ontario.)

The Ontario School of Osteopathy and Alternative Medicine

The Ontario School of Osteopathy and Alternative Medicine operates two campuses in the GTA—Markham and Mississauga. Graduates of the school are awarded the DO(MP) or "Diploma in Osteopathic Manual Practitioners"[sic] after successfully completing its "modular program, comprised of fourteen modules. Each module is three full days comprised of theory and clinical trainings."[140]

In its *2013-2014 Syllabus & Student Handbook*, the OSO's school director Dr. Mohsen Talani says in a message that "osteopathy is more than just a set of books; it is a way of looking at life. By being educated in osteopathy, you will change for the better as a human being. What you carry with you from this college will profoundly help improve other people's lives."

The handbook notes that the school "places a high value on its academic community and culture by fostering the development of an osteopathic learning organization."[141]

The OSO also offers "single Modules as Continuing Education Courses to add new Osteopathic techniques" to a person's practice.

Southern Ontario College of Osteopathy

Mississauga-based Southern Ontario College of Osteopathy offers a three-year program of study leading to a diploma in Osteopathy (Osteopathic Manipulative Practice). The college says on its website that its program "includes a total of 22 intense three-day thematic modules" that are carried over three years including eight weeks of individual clinical training, covering essential topics for osteopathic manipulative practice. Students graduate only after they have done clinical rotations, passed written, oral and practical examinations, and defended a thesis.[142]

The program covers manual osteopathy theory, clinical anatomy, physiology and biomechanics, review of major medical conditions, physical examination including osteopathic, neurologic and orthopedic assessment, medical imaging and the various osteopathic manual techniques.

Osteopathic College of Ontario

The Osteopathic College of Ontario (OCO) in Markham offers a three-year "Diplomate in Osteopathic Manipulative Theory & Practice" program that is tailored to "existing" health care practitioners. The main features of the program are thirteen "three-day quanta" given four times per year plus four individual weeks of individualized clinical training.[143]

The college is a partner with the Osteopathic Health & Wellness Institute in Parkesburg, PA, in running its program called an "International Diplomate Program" because it is concurrently offered in Switzerland, Japan, Hong Kong, Jordan, South Korea, and The Philippines.

The college says in a "question and answer" feature on its website, in terms of an "authority accredit(ing) this course," it is affiliated with the Ontario Federation of Osteopathic Professionals and The Society of Osteopaths of Canada and that when students complete the Diplomate program they are eligible for registration with either association.

London College of Osteopathy

The London College of Osteopathy offers several on-line osteopathy programs. Its "Associate Certificate in Osteopathy" takes about 150 hours to complete and consists of audio lectures, readings and videos. It is geared to healthcare and wellness professionals. The college also offers a "Certificate for Skin Care Specialists" which it says "enables skin care professionals to integrate specific osteopathic modalities into anti-aging and post surgical treatments."[144]

To make up for the omission of hands-on clinical practice in its programs, the college offers some of its graduates a supervised clinic in Toronto and Barcelona, Spain with a five-day tutorial.

Qualifications to Practise Osteopathic Medicine in Ontario in 2015

Required Qualifications

- Graduate of a college of osteopathic medicine accredited by the American Osteopathic Association and the Canadian Osteopathic Association
- Holder of Licentiateship from the Medical Council of Canada
- Successful completion of an internship with the College of Family Physicians of Canada or Royal College of Physicians and Surgeons of Canada.

Note: This list of qualifications may apply to all jurisdictions once each jurisdiction, with approval of its provincial or territorial government, passes enabling legislation for a "National Standard" for licensing medical doctors. (The registrars of the provincial and territorial medical regulatory authorities have signed an agreement in principle to introduce the standard which was developed by the Federation of Medical Regulatory Authorities of Canada.)

Qualifications to Practise as an Non-Physician Osteopath in 2015

Non-physician osteopathy is unregulated in Canada.

In the interest of public safety, the World Health Organization (WHO) has urged Canadian jurisdictions, since 2010, to adopt its benchmark standards of training for osteopaths.

Members of the Canadian Federation of Osteopaths adhere to the WHO benchmarks that include core competences such as a strong foundation in osteopathic history, philosophy, and approach to health care, and an understanding of the basic sciences within the context of the philosophy of osteopathy and the five models of structure-function.

Other core competencies that the directing and coordinating authority for health within the United Nations considers important:

- ability to form an appropriate differential diagnosis and treatment plan;
- an understanding of the mechanisms of action of manual therapeutic interventions and the biochemical, cellular and gross

anatomical response to therapy;

- ability to appraise medical and scientific literature critically and incorporate relevant information into clinical practice;
- competency in the palpatory and clinical skills necessary to diagnose dysfunction in the aforementioned systems and tissues of the body, with an emphasis on osteopathic diagnosis;
- competency in a broad range of skills of OMT;
- proficiency in physical examination and the interpretation of relevant tests and data, including diagnostic imaging and laboratory results;
- an understanding of the biomechanics of the human body including, but not limited to, the articular, fascial, muscular and fluid systems of the extremities, spine, head, pelvis, abdomen and torso;
- expertise in the diagnosis and OMT of neuromusculoskeletal disorders; and
- thorough knowledge of the indications for, and contraindications to, osteopathic treatment; a basic knowledge of commonly used traditional medicine and complementary/ alternative medicine techniques.

The WHO has also recommended that training curriculum include courses in Basic Science, Clinical Science, Osteopathic Science, Practical Skills, Osteopathic Skills, and Practical Supervised Clinical experience.

CHAPTER 17—OSTEOPATHY TODAY IN THE OTHER PROVINCES AND THE TERRITORIES

Governing the activities of osteopathic practitioners is a function performed by provincial and territorial governments.

There are two types of osteopathic practitioners: first, there are osteopaths who are generally described as "non-physician practitioners" of osteopathy. These osteopaths also have different occupational titles depending on the jurisdiction: in British Columbia, they are called "osteopathic practitioners," in Alberta, "osteopathic manual therapists," and in Nova Scotia, "osteopathic manual practitioners." It is estimated there are more than 2,000 of this class of osteopathic practitioners in Canada.

Second, there are the osteopathic physicians (also called DOs—doctors of osteopathic medicine) of which there are relatively few. In 2014, Ontario had the largest number with fewer than 50. The title "osteopath" is protected and controlled, in some provinces, like Nova Scotia, for example, by the respective regulatory medical authority.

Osteopathic physicians are regulated generally by provincial colleges of physicians and surgeons or health councils as in the case of the territories, depending on the regulations approved by their respective government. Like the health acts, these regulations are not uniform across the land.

In 2015, the manual osteopathic profession remains unregulated. On a daily basis, the practitioners operate under laws related to health care or business activities.

However, there are changes in progress in one province that, if carried to their logical conclusion, would affect many osteopathic manual practitioners in the coming years. The Quebec Office of Professions (Office des professions du Québec), a provincial advisory agency, has mandated a working group to develop draft recommendations that may lead to a future adoption of a regulatory framework by the Quebec government. The group began its deliberations in December 2014.

Alberta

In Alberta, Alberta Health Services (AHS) is responsible for the planning and delivery of health services in the province. A Board governs the activities of the AHS and reports to the Minister of Health and Wellness.

Osteopathic Physicians

The main statute and related regulations currently governing physicians, including osteopathic physicians in Alberta, are *The Health Professions Act* and *Regulation 350/2009* (the Physicians, Surgeons and Osteopaths Profession Regulation) and amendments in Alberta *Regulation 59/2012*.

In 1982, with regulatory approval from the provincial government, the College of Physicians and Surgeons of Alberta (CPSA) began registering osteopathic doctors as it does today. The college's requirement, since 1987, however, was that DOs had to graduate from "an accredited school of osteopathy." Later, in 2008, the college made it clear that the osteopathy degree had to be issued by an osteopathic school accredited by the American Osteopathic Association's (AOA) Commission on Osteopathic College Accreditation, according to Kelly Eby, a spokesperson for the CPSA.[145]

The Alberta medical regulatory authority has also signed off on an agreement in principle to adopt a national standard for licensing physicians. The document, *Standards for Medical Registration in Canada*, was developed by the Federation of Medical Regulatory Authorities of Canada (FMRAC).

The Alberta Medical Association, a group representing the province's physicians, has been on-side with the college's decisions. A doctor at the association's professional affairs section, said Alberta's doctors of osteopathic medicine are viewed "the same as regular physicians and . . . are governed by the CPSA." The doctor added, "there are very few in Alberta, to my knowledge."[146]

Osteopaths (called Osteopathic Manual Therapists in Alberta)

The most significant supply and service hub for the country's oil reserves and also known for its famous tourist centres such as Banff and Jasper, Alberta is starting to wake up to the value of manual osteopathy in keeping its four million residents healthy. Half of its population is located in Calgary and Edmonton and it is in the former city where one of Canada's largest single site locations of osteopathic manual therapists is found.

Intrinsi, founded in 2007 by British-trained osteopaths Ed Paget and his wife Lucille, employs five other osteopathic professionals who provide thousands of treatments each year at its south-west Calgary clinic.

Paget is also president of the Alberta Association of Osteopathic Manual Therapists (AAOMT) which has been formed to bring practitioners together. "Generally speaking, people work by themselves and the association is something that reminds them they are part of a profession," he said. The association which has more than 25 members, also provides them "with some camaraderie—sometimes there are meet-up education groups in Calgary and Edmonton so we can continue conversing with our colleagues."

"The association, more importantly, exists to educate the public about how osteopathic manual therapists can address the root causes of pain and what patients themselves can do to maintain the benefits of osteopathic treatments," Paget said.

The association president said he and the other officers of the association are committed to setting the standards of manual osteopathic practice in Alberta by approving candidates for membership who "meet or exceed the standards in osteopathic education as outlined by the World Health Organization (WHO) in 2010. This means that they will either have completed a four-year full-time degree course, similar to physiotherapists, or a part-time equivalent."[147]

The Canadian Federation of Osteopaths (CFO), of which the AAOMT is a member, says the Alberta group represents "a first step in the organization and regulation of manual practice osteopathic therapists" in the province.[148]

Osteopaths in Alberta are called "osteopathic manual therapists." The province's *Health Professions Act* grants protection of the titles "osteopathic practitioner" and "osteopath" to be used exclusively by osteopathic physicians.[149]

Looking forward, the AAOMT president said he is keeping an eye on developments in Quebec where the government is doing work that may lead to the province announcing a regulatory framework for the province's osteopathic manual practitioners. "A provincial standard of education is important," he said, "and Quebec may well set the standard that Alberta will likely follow." There are currently other osteopathic manual therapists practising in Alberta but they are not members because they don't meet our educational guidelines."

Paget also said he is looking forward to the day when osteopathic manual therapists in Alberta would be able to become a part of primary health care teams. He predicts that new continuing education requirements would have to be instituted so that osteopathic manual practitioners can pick up skill sets "similar to other professionals" in diagnosing illness.[150]

A fairly recent newcomer to osteopathic manual training in Alberta is the National Manual Osteopathic College (NMOC) located in Red Deer, the province's third most-populous city. It offers a 1526-hour "Manual Osteopathic Diploma" following a ten-month training program.

According to the college, the training objective is to "provide those working in a therapeutic environment with a set of additional evaluative and corrective techniques that will quickly and efficiently correct problems that current techniques are unable to address."[151]

The program consists of 13 two-day modules of classroom training, approximately 20-30 hours per week of self-directed learning, and 150 hours of clinical experience.

To help its graduates become registered osteopathic manual therapists, the college established the National Manual Osteopathic Society (NMOS).

British Columbia

In British Columbia, the Ministry of Health manages the health care system.

Osteopathic Physicians

To meet all of the requirements of the "full class of registration" with the College of Physicians and Surgeons of British Columbia, DOs need to have formal degrees in osteopathic medicine from a school or college accredited by the American Osteopathic Association. In addition, they must have completed the three-part comprehensive osteopathic medical licensing examinations administered by the United States National Board of Osteopathic Medical Examiners.

Additionally, for those osteopathic physicians with a special interest in musculoskeletal and manual medicine, a separate class of licensure for "osteopathic practice" is provided for in these bylaws. This class of registration is defined in section 2-13 of the bylaws made under the *Health Professions Act*.[152]

Under the bylaws of the College of Physicians and Surgeons of British

Columbia, United States national licensure examinations including COMLEX-USA, USMLE, FLEX, and NBME[153] are now recognized for full registration with the College.

Quoting Section 2-13 of the bylaws under the 2009 *Health Professions Act*, Susan Prins, a spokesperson for the college, said in an e-mail: "This specific class of registration permits a registrant to practise in the field of musculoskeletal medicine, primarily in the musculoskeletal system and associated conditions." The medical regulatory body's representative added that "osteopathic registrants may not practise primary care obstetrics or surgery."[154]

The college, in June 2013, signed an agreement in principle to implement a national standard for licensing medical doctors in its jurisdiction. The agreement was developed by the Federation of Medical Regulatory Authorities of Canada (FMRAC).

This common national standard was developed to satisfy the labour mobility provisions of the Agreement on Internal Trade (AIT), that promotes unrestricted mobility for medical doctors between provinces and the territories. In 2014, there were four DOs in the British Columbia college's records related to the "osteopathic class of registration."

Osteopaths (called Osteopathic Practitioners in British Columbia)

At her home-based office, Julie Brown reflects on how the osteopathic practitioner group she heads is evolving—and she likes it. The director of the Society for the Promotion of Manual Practice Osteopathy in Invermere, B.C., is pretty happy with the way things are going and she plans "to go step by step in moving forward and to let things unfold."[155]

With more than 50 members, the Society is moving forward with a focus on "building our bond as a group" while establishing relationships with stakeholders such as insurance companies and the Ministry of Health, and importantly, while "developing the processes to maintain the standards we have put in place," said Brown.

As the group tries to increase its membership over the coming years with a goal of 300, Brown is preoccupied not only with building her own practice at Osteohands but also working closely with the Society's executive board and members to "develop a good sense of who we are as a profession and as an organization."

Says Brown: "We are building a really positive culture. There are a lot of very good people in the profession [in B.C.] that are involved and I'd say we are very well supported by others in osteopathy across the country, through federal networks, through our own professional networks, even with the colleges [of manual osteopathy]—we're definitely growing a collaborative spirit."

As for attaining the group's membership target, considered by researchers to be the threshold that governments accept for regulatory review, it is not a tough goal, Brown surmises, considering the province is a favourite immigration destination point for manual osteopaths from Great Britain, Spain, France, Italy, Australia, and New Zealand.

The Society, which was incorporated in 2005 under the province's *Society Act*, allows for two membership classes under its bylaws: full members and student members. The group's aims include public education about osteopathy and being accountable through a professional code of conduct and its related components such as high ethical standards of practice, competency and practice rules, and ethical guidelines.

The Society is a member of the CFO (Canadian Federation of Osteopaths), a national association of provincial and territorial osteopathy groups, based in Quebec. Internationally, the provincial association is affiliated with the Chicago-based International Osteopathic Alliance whose mission is to further the practice of manual osteopathy and osteopathic medicine throughout the globe.

Manitoba

In Manitoba, the Department of Health, Healthy Living and Seniors is responsible for developing and administering the province's health care policies.

Osteopathic Physicians

Under the New Democratic provincial government of Gary Doer in 2003, the province approved *Regulation 25/2003*. This *Registration of Medical Practitioners Regulation* set out the qualifications for registration as a medical doctor in the province. As osteopathic physicians are graduates of foreign schools of medicine, they come under Section 11 (1)(b) of the province's *Medical Act*. Such graduates are required to pass "a screening process approved by Council" of the college.[156]

If doctors of osteopathic medicine apply for registration, they must have ". . . a degree from a school of osteopathic medicine in the United States of America approved by the American Association of Colleges of

Osteopathic Medicine," to be entered into the college's Educational Register, according to Marvin Giesbrecht, a lawyer with the corporate services department of the college.[157]

Like other provincial medical regulatory bodies, the college issues a licence to osteopathic medicine graduates provided they meet other requirements, including passing Part 1 and Part 2 of the Medical Council of Canada Qualifying Examination and successfully completing a residency.

The college is also a signatory to an agreement in principle developed by the FMRAC (Federation of Medical Regulatory Authorities of Canada) for the *Standards for Medical Registration in Canada*. This national standard for registering medical doctors was developed to support greater inter-jurisdictional mobility for them across the country.

**

In Manitoba, a parallel group of osteopathic medical practitioners has been organized by naturopath Dr. Paul Conyette from his Canadian Biologics offices in Winnipeg and Brandon. The group consists of "credentialed medical doctors who have graduated from World Health Organization (WHO)-recognized medical schools," said Conyette who, according to his biography once "completed Hospital rounds and emergency rotations at Brandon Hospital under Dr. M.J. Lau."[158]

"These medical doctors have also written and passed the Canadian MD exams—that is, the Medical Council of Canada Qualifying Examination. The only thing they are waiting for is to get a residency. But many of these smart men and women are not able to get one [at this time],"said Dr. Conyette.[159].

"So I'm heading up an association to allow them to get into the Canadian medical system. Eventually we want to apply for regulation in Manitoba. Our group is called the Manitoba Osteopathic Doctors Association (MODA). We call ourselves doctors of osteopathic manual sciences," he explained.

"My group is [made up of] strictly medical doctors who have had hospital training. We will also accept naturopathic doctors who have had hospital training as well," added Conyette, who is a multi-disciplinary health care services provider with a string of qualifications (TRT, MLT, BHSc, ND, DAc and IMD), including the NMD (naturopathic medical doctor) which in Arizona is also a physician's licence.[160]

Conyette draws a line between his group (doctors of osteopathic manual sciences) and the Canadian Osteopathic Association whose members are registered with provincial regulatory colleges of physicians and surgeons and territorial health councils.

(In 2014, there was no formal association of osteopathic manual practitioners in Manitoba although there is a "growing student association, which is in contact with the Canadian Federation of Osteopaths", a national association of provincial manual osteopath associations.)[161]

To join MODA, Conyette says "the criteria are that you have to be a medical doctor or a naturopathic doctor with one-year hospital training."

About the future, he has a vision of an organization from coast-to-coast. "We're going eventually to create a whole new national organization—a federation of doctors of osteopathic manual sciences in the provinces and territories who will have, eventually, MD or NMD hospital training and emergency medical training."

Conyette said his organization's members "will also have training in surgery, prescription writing, etc., not just manual medicine. Also, our doctors will be trained in herbalism, acupuncture, counselling, nutritional medicine . . . the whole ball of wax. We're not going to be just osteopathic manual practitioners. We will have a scope of practice that will be very broad."

Osteopaths

Austrian-born Florian Lassnig, a massage therapist and a final year osteopathic manual student at the Winnipeg branch of the Canadian College of Osteopathy, says that the demand for manual osteopathic services is growing but there is an insufficient number of trained manual osteopaths. "We can't fill it [the demand] yet. Even for the [manual osteopathy] students, most of us are fairly busy," said Lassnig who runs his clinic four days a week at Morden, a southern Manitoba city that was designated a "2008 Cultural Capital of Canada" with under 50,000 residents.

In 2014, there was no title protection in Manitoba for "osteopath," the website of the Canadian Federation of Osteopaths says.[162] This means osteopathic practitioners can call themselves osteopaths and practise under the "common law"(also known as case law or precedent, which is law developed by judges through decisions of courts and similar tribunals rather than through legislative statutes or executive branch action.)[163]

The City of Winnipeg is one of the Western Canada locations of The Collège d'Études Ostéopathiques de Montréal (the other is in British Columbia). The first set of graduates is expected to graduate in the latter part of the 2010s. The Canadian Federation of Osteopaths (CFO), which represents provincial associations of osteopathic practitioners, predicts an active Manitoba association of manual osteopaths would emerge and come into its fold.[164]

New Brunswick

In New Brunswick, the Ministry of Health oversees the health care system in the province.

Osteopathic Physicians

Like other Canadian jurisdictions, the College of Physicians and Surgeons of New Brunswick (CPSNB) recognizes the osteopathic degree issued by American Osteopathic Association-approved colleges of osteopathic medicine.

The college's registration and licensing regulation, known as Regulation No. 2, states that physicians may be eligible for registration with a "Defined, or Defined Locum, licence" if they have an osteopathic medical school degree approved by its governing council. The physicians would also have to meet other requirements such as being awarded a Licentiate by the Medical Council of Canada and successfully completing a residency.

Regulation No. 2 may also allow physicians not otherwise eligible for a licence to be registered and licensed with "Special" or "Special Locum" licence if they are graduates of a Council-approved osteopathic medical school and the licence is requested by a regional health authority for granting privileges to physicians. Such licences may also be issued if the request is made by a public department, agency, institution, commission, or similar authority for job objectives.

The college's regulation is in line with its earlier agreement in principle—with other provinces and the territories—to adopt the "Canadian Standard for Full Licensure" for physician registration and licensure which is a key element in the *Standards for Medical Registration in Canada* document developed by FMRAC (the Federation of Medical Regulatory Authorities of Canada).[165]

Osteopaths

Leading a small group of 16 osteopathic manual practitioners in New Brunswick, Pierrette Richer, president of the Association of Osteopaths of New Brunswick (l'Association des Ostéopathes du Nouveau-Brunswick) and her board of directors are forging ahead to build on the foundation laid by its founding president, who passed away in 2009.

The association is reviewing its by-laws, membership entry and practice standards to ensure they work to protect the public and is working closely with the Canadian Federation of Osteopaths because "we all have the same concerns about osteopathy."

Going into her fifth year as leader of the group, Richer speaks with unbridled energy about where she wants to take the association. Regulation of the profession by the government is not an immediate priority for the group, said Richer. The top priorities for the next few years include ensuring its rules on self-regulation as a professional group are enforced in order for the public to obtain top-notch service from its members who serve tens of thousands of English-speaking and Francophone osteopathic patients in the province of 750,000 residents.

She remarked that her energy comes from the residents' trust in what her members do for a living. "The people recognize us and they support us," said Richer. "And that's very nice."

Newfoundland and Labrador

In Newfoundland and Labrador, the Ministry of Health and Community Services oversees the development and delivery of health care services in the province.

Osteopathic Physicians

Graduates of U.S. osteopathic medicine colleges are recognized by the College of Physicians and Surgeons of Newfoundland and Labrador as being eligible to practise medicine in Newfoundland and Labrador, once they meet other requirements. This has been a relatively new development.

In 2011, the Progressive Conservative government of Kathy Dunderdale approved significant changes to the province's *Medical Act*, 2011. Subsequently, it passed the Medical Board regulations on physician registration and licensure. In June 2013, the College of Physicians and Surgeons of Newfoundland and Labrador signed an agreement in principle with the other provincial medical regulatory colleges and the territorial health councils to introduce a national standard for physician licensure proposed by the Federation of Medical Regulatory Authorities of Canada.

Under the new regulations, physicians applying for the first time for full licensure will be required to have graduated from an acceptable allopathic or osteopathic medical school; be awarded a Licentiate of the Medical Council of Canada; have completed a post-graduate training program in allopathic medicine; and have successfully completed a residency through the College of Family Physicians of Canada or the Royal College of Physicians and Surgeons of Canada.

Like the eligibility criteria to obtain a licence in other jurisdictions, osteopathic physicians must satisfy other screening requirements.

Osteopaths

In 2015, there is at least one osteopath in Newfoundland and Labrador. For the past 12 years, Michael Eddy, owner of Michael Eddy Osteopathy in St. John's, has been emphasizing cranial osteopathy and "BioDynamics" in his practice. He also works at The Wellness Centre, a 14-person team of health professionals, including a physician, a clinical sexologist, a psychologist, and a a massage therapist.

A provincial association of osteopaths does not exist. If and when a larger number of osteopathic practitioners do establish practices and attain a critical mass, they can apply, as a group, to the Minister of Health and Community Services for regulatory status.

Northwest Territories

In the Northwest Territories, the Department of Health and Social Services oversees the delivery of the health care services. The department is responsible for legislation governing twelve health professions, including physicians, and these are covered by eleven different Acts.

Osteopathic Physicians

When Samantha Van Genne wrote in an August 26, 2014 e-mail that " . . . we are a small jurisdiction [and] we are entirely reliant on provincial assessment," the Northwest Territories registrar of professional licensing added that "our legislation only recognized family physicians or Royal College [of Physicians and Surgeons of Canada] specialists for licensure as a physician.

"Should an American physician seek licensure here who has the medical degree in osteopathic medicine but has completed certification with [the] Royal College we would consider this if he /she is on the full physician register in Ontario," she explained.[166]

The licensing and credentialing processes now in place to assess licence applications by doctors of osteopathic medicine are changing. The Medical Registration Committee of the Northwest Territories, which is responsible for issuing licences to practise medicine, is working to align its mechanisms so it can adjust to the territory's plan to introduce a national standard for full licensure.

The Northwest Territories' health council is a signatory to an agreement in principle, developed by the Federation of Medical Regulatory Authorities of Canada (FMRAC), to implement FMRAC's *Standards for Medical Registration in Canada*.

Osteopaths

Like other Canadian jurisdictions, osteopathy is unregulated in the second largest of the three territories. Internet searches undertaken by the authors in 2014 revealed there were no osteopaths among its 43,000 residents. If and when practitioners do establish practices and have attained a critical mass in numbers, they can apply, as a group, to the Minister of Health and Social Services for regulatory status.

Nova Scotia

In Nova Scotia, the Department of Health and Wellness oversees the health care system in the province.

Osteopathic Physicians

In 2011, the New Democratic government of Darrell Dexter passed the *Medical Act* requiring the College of Physicians and Surgeons of Nova Scotia to regulate the practice of medicine and to keep registers of those persons who qualify for registration.

Introducing the legislation, Health Minister Maureen Macdonald told the Legislative Assembly that it would ". . . develop processes to permit non-physicians to take on certain aspects of the practice of medicine."[167]

Supporting the bill, MLA Diana Whalen, who is, in 2015, is the Deputy Premier of Nova Scotia, said, referring to doctors of osteopathy:

They have a slightly different training but it does cover all of the bases for our

*medical training. This bill will allow them to be fully recognized to practice here
in our province. That aligns us as well, I believe, with other jurisdictions in
Canada so that we've got better mobility and we become, again, in sync with our
neighbouring provinces and recognizing that these doctors, who are trained in the
United States, may have a different approach to some of the work they do, as
physicians, but they certainly have all of the solid grounding that we provide in
Nova Scotia.168*

The College of Physicians and Surgeons of Nova Scotia recognizes a
degree in osteopathic medicine (DO) from U.S. osteopathic medical
schools accredited by the American Osteopathic Association as equivalent
to a medical doctor, according to the registrar of the college.[169] The
statutory basis of that statement is Sections 22(3) of the Act which states
in part, ". . . no person shall use the title "Doctor of Osteopathy" or
abbreviations or derivations thereof or the title "Osteopathic Physician"
unless that person (a) is a medical practitioner; and (b) holds an
osteopathic medical degree from a school approved by the Council for
this purpose."

"Of course, the requirements for a Full licence," the registrar notes,
". . . are that candidates hold the LMCC (Licentiate of the Medical Council
of Canada) and certification in either Family Medicine from the College
of Family Physicians of Canada or in a speciality from the Royal College
of Physicians and Surgeons of Canada.

"Provided an applicant with a DO has appropriate post graduate
training and certification and has successfully passed all three steps of the
USMLE (United States Medical Licensing Examination) or the
COMLEX-USA (Comprehensive Osteopathic Medical Licensing
Examination), they would be eligible for a Defined licence in Nova
Scotia," the letter said.

The registrar of the College of Physicians and Surgeons of Nova Scotia
has signed an agreement in principle to implement FMRAC's (the
Federation of Medical Regulatory Authorities of Canada) Standards for
Medical Registration in Canada.[170]

Osteopaths (called Osteopathic Manual Practitioners in Nova Scotia)

In 2006, osteopathic manual practitioners formed a group called the Nova
Scotia Association of osteopaths (NSAO). The association is currently
working with the College of Physicians and Surgeons of Nova Scotia and

the current and past provincial government officials to seek regulation for non-physician osteopaths. According to the association, this may facilitate future legislation that will affect those who practise osteopathic manual therapy.[171]

In the future, should the NSAO obtain statutory regulation for the province's osteopathic manual practitioners—referred to as osteopaths in most other Canadian jurisdictions—*Regulation 61/2014,* approved under the province's 2012 *Regulated Health Professions Network Act,* can potentially impact its members.

The 2012 legislation attempts, among other objectives, to increase collaboration among "Network" members—that is, regulated health professions.

According to the College of Nurses of Nova Scotia, the Network can be used "as a forum for communication, to share resources and expertise, collaborate on projects and identify common issues and concerns," the nurses' regulatory agency wrote. "In Nova Scotia, our health care system is continuing to move towards collaborative inter-professional care teams. These teams enable health professionals to work together in the most effective and efficient way so that they can produce the best health outcomes for clients.[172]

According to the regulation, a "regulated health profession" is a Network member whose scope of practice is defined in its governing statute and has standards of practice and a code of ethics in place.

The legislation also states that Network membership is contingent upon the governing statute of the profession being in effect. As well, the profession must have established a college, association, board or other entity to regulate the profession in the public interest, and has set out membership criteria.

In setting out established criteria for a regulation health profession in Nova Scotia , the government has followed the standards established in Ontario and other provinces in defining a regulated profession. Other criteria include: the regulated profession must have developed investigatory, adjudicatory and resolution processes regarding public complaints against members.

Nunavut

In Nunavut, the Department of Health and Social Services coordinates the delivery of health care to the territory's residents. Its mission is "to promote, protect and enhance the health and well-being of all

Nunavummiut, incorporating Inuit Qaujimajatuqangit [an Inuktitut phrase that is often translated as 'Inuit traditional knowledge,' 'Inuit traditional institutions,' or even 'Inuit traditional technology'] at all levels of service delivery and design."[173]

Osteopathic Physicians

Nunavut's Department of Health and Social Services has long been welcoming medical doctors to practise medicine in the territory as part of its "Flying Doctors Service." According to an Internet notice, "this is a truly unique opportunity to experience rich Inuit culture, breathtaking scenery and a change of pace."

The department warns "there are no roads into Nunavut from other parts of Canada, nor between any of our 25 communities. General travel is by air, although it is possible to travel by boat, snow machine or dog team."[174]

Doctors of osteopathic medicine must be licensed by the Medical Registration Committee of Nunavut, which meets every two weeks to consider applications. To be eligible, they must have passed Canadian medical examinations (that is, Parts 1 and 2 of the Medical Council of Canada Qualifying Examinations and completed a residency program) and have a letter of good standing.[175]

Like other territories and the provinces, Nunavut has signed an agreement in principle with the Federation of Medical Regulatory Authorities of Canada to implement a national standard for licensing medical doctors.

Osteopaths

Osteopathy is unregulated in Nunavut, the largest of the three territories. There are apparently no osteopaths practising among its 36,600 residents (2014) who live in 26 settlement areas. If and when practitioners do establish practices and have attained a critical mass in numbers, they can apply, as a group, to the Minister of Health and Social Services for regulation of the profession.

Prince Edward Island

In Prince Edward Island, the Department of Health and Wellness is responsible for the delivery of health care services.

Osteopathic Physicians

The province currently regulates 16 health professions, including medical doctors, through 14 statutes and regulations.

On May 1, 2014, the Liberal government of Robert Ghiz approved regulations under the *Medical Act* that gave title protection to doctors of osteopaths, or who are graduates of osteopathic colleges recognized by the American Osteopathic Association's system of accreditation.[176]

As with all Canadian provincial and territorial jurisdictions, doctors of osteopathic medicine are eligible for licensing as medical doctors once they are licentiates of the Medical Council of Canada and hold a certificate from the Royal College of Physicians and Surgeons of Canada or the College of Family Physicians of Canada.

The provincial medical authority had signed an agreement in principle to introduce a national standard for licensing medical doctors. The agreement was developed by the Federation of Medical Regulatory Authorities of Canada.

On May 1, 2014,.the Council of the College of Physicians and Surgeons of Prince Edward Island issued revised college regulations in which the American Osteopathic Association is referenced.[177]

Osteopaths

There are several practising osteopaths in the province but they have not yet formed an association to make representations to the government for regulation.

In August 2012, Doug Currie, Minister of Health and Wellness, proposed, in a consultation document, new umbrella health professions legislation with the goal of regulating several new health professional groups within the province. According to the minister, the purpose of umbrella health professions legislation "is to provide consistency in the core components of professional legislation."

"[T]he creation of consistent administrative, complaint, and discipline processes ensures fairness, transparency, and accountability to the public and to the health professions alike," Currie added.

The consultation included the proposed draft legislation regarding unregulated professions (osteopaths apparently qualify as they are unregulated).

Upon receiving an application from an organization that represents the majority of the members of a health profession in the province, the

Minister will refer the application to the Advisory Council to investigate and advise whether it is in the public interest to regulate the profession, the consultation document says.

Membership in the various health professions range from four to over 600 practitioners. The minister said that health professions as a result do not have the human or financial resources to self-regulate.[178]

Saskatchewan

In Saskatchewan, the Ministry of Health and the Minister Responsible for Rural and Remote Health oversee the delivery of health care services. The ministry is responsible for overseeing the activities of 26 health professions including physicians, naturopathic practitioners and chiropractors. (Part of its licensing and regulatory mandate is to make them accountable through various means, including requiring "the health professional to be registered and licensed to use the title of the profession and perform certain services.")[179]

Osteopathic Physicians

The College of Physicians and Surgeons of Saskatchewan governs physicians under the *Medical Professions Act* (MPA) enacted in 1981 and its bylaws made under the MPA.

The college accepts the qualifications of osteopathic doctors provided they meet other screening requirements. According to the college's regulatory bylaw No. 2.3(c)(iv), '[it] is a non-exemptible standard and qualification for registration and a licence to practise medicine that an applicant have a degree in medicine that was at the time the degree was awarded . . . a Doctor of Osteopathic Medicine degree from a school in the United States accredited by the American Osteopathic Association Commission on Osteopathic College Accreditation."[180]

The change is the result of the province's decision to align its physician registration standard with a national one prepared by the Federation of Medical Regulatory Authorities of Canada (FMRAC). Prior to June 2013 when the regulatory medical college signed an agreement in principle with the FMRAC, DOs were unable to obtain licensure with the college. "That was an issue which was discussed with the provincial government for several years, with the College suggesting that the legislation be amended to remove the requirement that a physician have a medical degree (as opposed to a DO degree) in order to be licensed," wrote a college spokesperson.[181]

"The first change occurred in 2010 when the government passed an amendment to the Act, the effect of which was to permit physicians with a D.O degree who had the LMCC and were licensed in another province to be licensed in Saskatchewan.

"The next amendment occurred in 2014 to remove the requirements for licensure from the Act and allow the College to adopt registration standards in bylaw," the college's associate registrar said.[182]

Osteopaths

Like Violet Clara McNaughton, the influential first president of the Women Grain Growers, who spearheaded drives for more nurses, doctors, and hospitals in all-rural Saskatchewan in 1914 , present-day Saskatchewanian Barbara Schultze is determined to get health-care workers from outside the province and Europe to set up shop inside the Bread Basket of Canada.

"I have put the word out to people to let them know there is a great demand in Saskatchewan for osteopathic manual practitioners," said Schultze, owner of the Élan Osteopathic Clinic in Regina and first president of the Saskatchewan Association of Osteopaths (SAO). "If qualified manual osteopaths want to come, they will be most welcome."[183]

Her survey of the market, based on her daily practice since 2001, reveals that manual osteopathy "is well accepted." "People are very curious. [Although] they don't exactly know what it is. They know it by the results," she says.

"People are accustomed to chiropractic and physiotherapy but a lot of things aren't addressed in those professions," Schultze notes. "Sometimes people reach a plateau where they are not getting the [health- care] answers they need, and they end up here. A lot of it is that people are looking for a more in-depth form of treatment."

An experienced advocate for registered massage therapists while a director of the Massage Therapist Association of Saskatchewan that has been lobbying the provincial government for regulatory status, Schultze is confident about the future for the fledging association she heads.

At the beginning of 2015, the SAO's membership roll stands at less than half a dozen. But that doesn't daunt Schultze, "Like everything else, you start at the beginning and go through the process," she said. "It's going to be a fairly long process in our province," she added.

In the meantime, the SAO is not resting on its laurels. It is encouraging

Saskatchewanians in the health care field to take a multi-year diploma course in osteopathic manual therapy.

As the SAO is committed to setting the standards of manual osteopathic practice in the province, Schultze has been collaborating with the Canadian Federation of Osteopaths, to develop a draft set of bylaws and a code of ethics. Entry-to-membership criteria are already in place and they include full members meeting or exceeding the benchmark guidelines for osteopathic education as outlined by the *Benchmarks for Training in Osteopathy* developed in 2010 by the World Health Organization (WHO).

This kind of non-governmental self-regulation is necessary, Schultze says, as "without some kind of regulation it would leave the field wide open for anybody to come in and claim to be an osteopath."

Yukon

In the Yukon, the Department of Health and Social Services oversees the delivery of health care services. However, under the *Medical Profession Act*, the Yukon Medical Council is responsible for regulating the practice of medicine and medical care provided by licensed physicians in the Yukon.[184]

Osteopathic Physicians

All physicians wishing to practise medicine in the Yukon must be a Licentiate of the Medical Council of Canada and hold a certificate of fellowship from the Royal College of Physicians and Surgeons of Canada or the College of Family Physicians of Canada, or hold a current Full licence in another province or territory of Canada that is a party to the Agreement on Internal Trade, according to the Yukon Medical Council's website.[185]

Karen Lincoln, the council's coordinator for professional licensing and regulatory affairs said, "Osteopaths are not regulated in Yukon, therefore licensure is not provided."[186]

But, like the other territories and the provinces, Yukon had signed, in June 2013, an agreement in principle with the Federation of Medical Regulatory Authorities of Canada to implement a national standard for licensing medical doctors.

Osteopaths

There is no regulation of osteopathy is the Yukon. Apparently, there are
no active practices set up in this territory to provide manual treatments.
At a later date, when practitioners have attained a critical mass in numbers,
they can apply, as a group, to the Minister of Health and Social Services
for regulation of the profession.

CHAPTER 18—ARE ONTARIO'S OSTEOPATHS 'REGULATION-READY?'

The Present Picture of a Disunited Profession

Leaning back on a couch in his cavernous office surrounded by dozens of healing arts diplomas, Dr. Sohrab Khoshbin remarked in the autumn of 2014 that he didn't understand why the eight professional groups representing Ontario's osteopathic manual practitioners have so far been unable to promote, as one association, manual osteopathy as a form of complementary health care.

"That's what I . . . always actually [did] . . . call the other associations . . . to gather together and make one association that is so strong," claimed Khoshbin, president of the Ontario Association of Osteopathy and Natural Medicine, one of the eight practitioner group.[187]

The single association idea suggested by the Iranian-educated holder of a doctorate degree in chemistry has not been lost on British Columbia – based Gail Abernethy, president of the Canadian Federation of Osteopaths (CFO), which represents the provincial and territorial manual osteopathic associations at a national and international level. Said Abernethy in a January 2015 interview: "We would be happy if all the suitably qualified people in Ontario got together and form one association."[188]

(The eight Ontario osteopathy advocacy groups the authors identified online at the beginning of 2015, using the Google Web search engine, are: the Ontario Association of Osteopathic Manual Practitioners (OAO); the Ontario Federation of Osteopathic Professionals (OFOP); the Ontario Osteopathic and Alternative Medicine Association (OOAMA); the Ontario Association of Osteopathy and Natural Medicine (OAONM)); the Ontario Osteopathic Association (OOA); the Ontario College of Osteopathic Rehabilitation Sciences (OCORS); the Ontario Council of Drugless Osteopathy (OCDO); and The International Osteopathic Association (IOA).)

The CFO's position about being "suitably qualified" is clear and unambiguous but a move to join the national body will be fraught with a major challenge for all the groups—except the OAO, which is already a member.

Because the CFO adopted the World Health Organization's (WHO's) training benchmarks for osteopathy, each *individual* member of the other associations would have to meet the WHO's educational requirements. A cursory review of the other seven groups' websites seems to indicate not all individual members conform to the international body's benchmarks.

As they all strive towards the same goal—presumably to get the ear of the provincial government—osteopathic observers say there is a lack of unity—another challenge—among the groups that speak for more than 800 Ontario practising osteopathic manual practitioners, and speculate as to why.

Pressure group politics expert, Paul Pross, Professor Emeritus at Nova Scotia's Dalhousie University, explains why there is a silent zone among the organizations: "The people who see themselves as genuine professionals do not want to have too much to do with the people who they see as amateurs and even perhaps as wonky, even crazy."

"Those people [the amateurs] in the eyes of would-be professionals are people who would be seen as not credible by government and by the other health professionals who would be asked to advise as to whether [the former] should be [part of the] profession," said Pross.

The retired professor, who continues to publish pieces on group politics, also points to the element of direct and indirect competition playing out as each group tries to develop a powerful advantage over the others. "Groups of people who are in the same line of work tend to sometimes be rivals as well as colleagues," he added.[189]

Dr. Jillian Kohler, director of global health at the University of Toronto's Munk School of Global Affairs, agrees with Pross: "[With these groups] there's going to be territorial and turf wars between them. Some are probably going to perceive they are more legitimate than the other groups."[190]

On the outcome of these "wars," says Kohler, "there's going to be winners and losers. Some of the groups are going to gain from it [a regulatory move by the government] and some are going to lose. The question is who is more likely to gain from being regulated . . . It might either create more restrictions on what they can do [or] they might have to be more qualified." Winning is obviously important for the associations and Pross adds that the more mature ones "are anxious not to see those rights and privileges [associated with government recognition] denied simply because they are associated with groups that are not credible."

Just by looking at their mission statements, it is evident that the groups are all shooting at the same target. Here are a few examples:

- A mission of the Ontario Federation of Osteopathic Professionals is "to work closely with [the] Ministry of Health in order to regulate osteopathic manual practice in Ontario."[191]

- The Ontario College of Osteopathic Rehabilitation Sciences, says its mission is to provide "policy input as a complement to the existing provincial legislation guiding the manual osteopathy profession in Ontario and all other related practices . . . ."[192]

- A key objective of one of the largest groups, the Ontario Association of Osteopathic Manual Practitioners, is "to seek support in Ontario for the enactment of legislation by government to regulate osteopathy by non-physician practitioners of osteopathy in Ontario, under the *Regulated Health Professions Act (1991)* or otherwise; and to make representation and submissions to the Minister of Health and Long-Term Care, the Health Professions Regulatory Advisory Council or HPRAC, the Government of Ontario and others for the enactment of such legislation.[193]

- "IOA [International Osteopathic Association] provides policy input as a complement to the existing national and international legislation guiding the manual osteopathy profession and all other related practices," says the Toronto-based IOA on its website.[194]

The polarized environment has created an atmosphere of suspicion is attitude has extended beyond the groups and schools –even to the point that some of them ignore or refuse invitations to be interviewed. In one case one school laid down unacceptable conditions just to be interviewed.[195]

Commenting on the political skills of the groups, Patricia L. O'Reilly, a Ryerson University political scientist who has done extensive research on health profession politics in the 1980s in Ontario, wrote the authors in an e-mail: "I have no knowledge whatsoever of the osteopaths' knowledge of the political system, so I cannot speak to their abilities. However, you will see in my work that I found considerable disparity among the health practitioner groups with regard to their knowledge of the political system and thus their ability to lobby effectively."[196]

"Many of them would have benefited from a Politics 101 course," O'Reilly suggested.

When further asked why the groups threw cold water on the authors' requests for an interview, she wrote: "I have no idea why some groups would not be responding to you. Your conjecture would be as good as mine. You could ask them."[197]

Setting the Stage for a Brighter Picture on the Horizon

Political scientists already know a lot about how governments go about deciding what particular health policies to adopt and what they will put on the backburner.

In a 2008 study, Patrick Fafard, social sciences professor at Ottawa University found ways to develop "healthy public policy." He wrote there were strategies that advocacy groups, what he called "public health actors" such as "policy advocates, lobbyists, decision-makers, journalists, public servants, and individual politicians," can adopt to get what they want."[198]

When there is a great amount of "scientific evidence" available, it would have very strong influence in health decisions, the study said. Research and knowledge transfer were also found to be important but they ended up being "not the full story." The professor also found that the positive effect of scientific evidence varied because it depended on the stage the policy-makers were at when decisions were being made.

Those who want to create an "enabling environment" for regulation to happen, would have to engage in strategic actions to create political debate and appeal to its health-care agenda, observers note.[199]

To the mix of Fafard's points, interest groups may consider what Dr. Joanne P. Boase has had to say about reaching out to government. They can use "sophisticated pressure group tactics.[which].can be highly effective as a surrogate for medical recognition." Boase, Professor Emeritus at the University of Windsor, knows quite a bit about getting a high public profile; she conducted many studies on government-group relationships in Ontario's health-care sector in the 1980s.[200]

In the meantime, the Ontario Association of Osteopathic Manual Practitioners is forging ahead with its attempts to gain attention. Elizabeth Leach, executive director of the association, said: "We have a plan . . .[and] we would be working on a strategy that we need to develop . . . in order to make a submission [to the government]. It's important for us to know what the requirements are and to determine whether it's the right time."[201]

The appropriate time is hard to determine.

And timing may depend on many factors, such as ongoing pressures to reduce the estimated provincial yearly health budget (in 2014 it was about

$50-billion) which absorbs more than 45% of the provincial budget. In speaking with osteopaths across Canada, the authors heard the claim often that osteopathy, by virtue of the value it delivers, can reduce health costs.

Riding Out the Current Lows with PR Lessons

It's been 18 years since former University of Ohio professor and octogenarian Hugh M. Culbertson and two colleagues wrote about how the U.S. osteopathic physician community had been strategically using public relations to overcome its challenges with the American Medical Association. Their 1993 book chapter on osteopathy public relations cast the U.S. osteopaths as the legendary "David" up against "Goliath," the powerful American Medical Association. David won, of course. A key point they raised is that winning over Herculean difficulties is often about relationships and building these while deploying strategic public relations.[202]

But first, what exactly is public relations?

In 2010, Culbertson described it well in another document. "Public relations, while often viewed as concerned primarily with persuasion (behaviour and/or attitude change), also focuses heavily on maintaining and building what clients and various stakeholders regard as favourable relationships."[203]

Some activities he suggested that can be implemented, depending on the context, to generate a buzz, (that is, healthy debate and positive responses from public policymakers and analysts) include:

- strengthen the training of practitioners in patient and public relations;
- produce visual media and readable brochures that present the osteopathy story;
- encourage practitioners to discuss patient communication with other health-care professionals;
- develop and market media features for practitioners about the long, slow, discouraging process of preventing and curing health-care problems;
- distribute media releases;
- provide training materials to practitioners;
- create informative brochures and videos for patients, showing practitioner and patient working together to deal with health problems;

- create brochures and videos for patients emphasizing patient responsibility and that "payment must come from somewhere";
- encourage osteopaths to become active in their communities, such as speaking to civic groups, and establishing physical fitness groups;
- take part in talk shows, write health columns in newspapers, put brochures in lobbies, and identify other channels to educate people on osteopathy;
- devise estimates, however rough, of costs, benefits, and savings connected with wellness and treatment linked to osteopathy; and
- develop analyses (perhaps looking in-depth at a broad range of specific cases) to clarify the human implications and decision-making dynamics, and of ways in which health-care as a whole would save money. Such analyses would attempt to assess how much money could be saved.

In the final analysis, experts in the art of lobbying and public relations encourage groups to make sure they strategically appeal to the value of the "public interest" in order to advance their professional concerns. They say the groups would have to address specific questions of themselves such as:

1) How do other health professions currently perceive them (and their practices as osteopathic manual practitioners) as they deliver health care to the community?
2) As future regulated professionals, are they now qualified and able to adhere to a proper standard that serves and protects the public?
3) What are their standards of professional practice, knowledge, skills, and professional ethics?

Osteopathy's Promising Future Lies in Canada

Given the apparent animosity in the Ontario osteopathy scene, the biblical injunction, "Peace be upon you . . . !" may be indicated. At least, osteopathic physician Vermont-based Steve Paulus, D.O., thinks so. An occasional facilitator in workshops at Ontario and Quebec manual osteopathy schools, Paulus has become well known since 2010 for his plea on the Internet, to osteopathic professionals around the world and across osteopathic streams to reflect deeper on their relationships with one another. Why? Because, according to him, "I'm tired of fighting; aren't you?"

In his Internet piece, "Undivided: Accepting Diversity within the

Osteopathic Profession," he uses anaphora—repetition of the same phrase—to emphasize and unify his message to Canadian, American, European, Australian and British osteopaths in both streams of osteopathy.

It is time for the allopathically oriented [oriented towards conventional medical practice] Osteopathic Physicians who don't utilize Osteopathic Manipulation to stop denigrating the American DOs who use OMT and integrate Osteopathic philosophy into their practices.

It is time for the DOs who use OMT on a regular basis to accept the value of those Osteopathic Physicians who practice exclusively allopathic medicine.

It is time for the Cranial Osteopaths to stop looking down upon the DOs who regularly use high velocity low amplitude methods or other more physical, direct action Osteopathic manipulative techniques.

It is time for the mechanically oriented DOs to stop ridiculing the Osteopaths who utilize a non-mechanical or a non-material Osteopathic approach.

It is time for those who want to call DOs Osteopathic Physicians to stop deriding the DOs who call themselves Osteopaths. It is time for the American DOs to stop belittling the British DOs, the other European DOs, Australian DOs, New Zealand DOs, Canadian DOs, and all of the non-American DOs who carry the torch of Osteopathy with passion and courage.

It is time for the British DOs to stop mocking the Canadian DOs. It is time for the various factions of European DOs to stop fighting and start uniting. It is time for the Australian and British DOs to stop claiming that they practice in alignment with A. T. Still's true teachings and the Osteopathically oriented American DOs don't.

It is time for DOs to stop patronizing the MD or Dentist who has sincerely embarked upon the study of Osteopathy. It is time to stop the international Osteopathic civil war and bring our energies together to do what we all do best— to care for people who need our help.

It is time for one group or one person to stop saying that they own the truth and that everyone else is wrong.

It is time . . . .[204]

Asked why he went public with his "It Is Time" campaign, Paulus, who has established a digital Osteopathic Public Library for the benefit of practitioners, told this book's authors that from his vantage point as a historian, osteopaths of all stripes will eventually tone down their current negative rhetoric. And, he predicted, it would only be a matter of time before they will be better integrated into the health-care system around the world.

Paulus said he wanted to remind Canada and the rest of the world what Dr. Viola M. Frymann once told him, as part of an audience of 150 DOs in a hotel several years ago: "The future of osteopathy will be in Canada and the rest of the world."[205]

What a Future Ontario Regulatory Initiative Might Look Like

A Registration Act, when passed into law in a provincial parliament, is essentially legislation that confers authority to a body to govern the affairs of a group of practitioners. On its proclamation by the Lieutenant-Governor of Ontario, the body would be classified as a "health regulatory college" as in the case of any health profession.

The *Regulated Health Professions Act (1991)*, under which the regulatory body would operate, includes a "schedule" called the Health Professions Procedural Code that sets out details of its legal and operational requirements.

The requirements would likely include the creation of a council of professional members and members of the general public to establish the college's mandate and manage the activities of the professionals

Key activities of the college would likely include the issuing of licences to eligible practitioners based on entry-to-practise standards, a code of ethics, practice guidelines, quality assurance programs, regulations regarding professional misconduct, and practitioner requirements for continuing education.

The formal beginning of such legislation in Ontario may be a "Ministerial Referral." This occurs when the Minister of Health and Long-Term Care is tasked with considering the regulation of a health profession.

In a referral, the Health Professions Regulatory Advisory Council (HPRAC), a consulting health policy agency at arm's length from the Ministry of Health and Long-Term Care, would lead the work of researching the profession and preparing a report for the minister.

The council is usually expected to cast a wide net to capture what it calls "knowledgeable information and comment from members of the public, community organizations, interest groups, health professional regulatory colleges and associations," and also conducts other extensive research. The minister would likely obtain a great array of "evidence-informed advice" from this process.

The information gathered would, in all likelihood, include reviews of literature on the profession: "jurisprudential and jurisdiction" reviews; that is, analyses of both the legislation/case law surrounding the profession's practices, and how other jurisdictions in the world regulate it.

Should the minister decide, based on the council's recommendations, that an unregulated health profession, such as manual osteopathy, should be regulated, the final outcome would usually be the enabling of legislation under the *Regulated Health Professions Act, 1991* (HRPA).

As of April 1, 2015, three other health professions were being reviewed in this "referral" pipeline: chiropody and podiatry, diagnostic sonographers, and paramedics.

Appendix 1—Select Milestones in Osteopathy and Medicine

1839 - College of Physicians and Surgeons of Upper Canada (now Ontario) is formed, but its incorporating Act is disallowed in 1840.

1847 - Establishment of the American Medical Association (AMA) in direct response to the rise of homeopaths and eclectics practitioners.

1847 - College of Physicians and Surgeons of Lower Canada (now Quebec) is established.

1859 - Ontario's first practising homeopath petitions the Legislative Assembly of Upper Canada (now Ontario) to recognize homeopathy.

1865 - *Medical Act* establishes medical licensure and educational standards in Western Canada.

1866 - College of Physicians and Surgeons of Ontario (CPSO) is established.

1867 - Canadian Medical Association (CMA) is established.

1871 - College of Physicians and Surgeons of Manitoba (CPSM) is established.

1874 - *Upper Canada Act* establishes strict regulation against unlicensed or "irregular" medical practitioners, such as doctors of osteopathy.

1875 - College of Physicians and Surgeons of Ontario appoints a prosecutor to challenge complementary and alternative health practitioners.

1885 - Dr. Andrew T. Still announces "Osteopathy" to be the name of the principles and practices of non-allopathic medicine he pioneered.

1890s - Doctors of Osteopathy attain limited medical practice rights in the U.S., and Dr. Andrew Taylor Still establishes an osteopathic college at Kirksville, Missouri.

1892 - First osteopathic medical school opens in Kirksville, Missouri.

1898 - Robert B. Henderson, Ontario's first osteopath sets up a practice in Toronto. (A turn-of-the 20th century author Emmons R. Booth, however, claimed that Dr. H.L. Spangler introduced osteopathy into Canada when he set up a practice at St. Johns, New Brunswick. Source: Emmons Rutledge Booth. *History of Osteopathy and Twentieth Century Medical Practice*. Cincinatti: Jennings and Graham, 1905, p.70.)

1899 - The first doctor of osteopathy arrives in Manitoba.

1901 - American Osteopathic Association is founded following the existence of a dozen of osteopathy schools in the U.S.

1903 - The first doctor of osteopathy arrives in Alberta.

1906 - Alberta College of Physicians and Surgeons is established.

1909 (circa) - First three doctors of osteopathy arrive in British Columbia.

1909 - *Medical Act* passed by the British Columbia government and it mentions chiropractic, naturopathy and osteopathy.

1910 - Osteopathic groups present *Bill 47* to "Incorporate the Osteopathic College of Ontario." (The Bill was later withdrawn.).

1910 - The *Flexner Report,* also called Carnegie Foundation Bulletin Number Four, prepared by Abraham Flexner, recommends reforms in medical education in the U.S. and Canada.

1910 - Dr. Andrew T. Still, founder of Osteopathy, publishes *Osteopathy Research and Practice.*

1912 - Passage of the Canada *Medical Act* unifies allopathic medical education across Canada.

1912 - Medical Council of Canada is established to create a uniform system and standards for physician assessment and practice for the country.

1913 - Manitoba Osteopathic Association is established.

1913 - *Osteopathy Act* is enacted in Saskatchewan, making it the first official board for registration and examination of osteopaths outside of the United States.

1917 - On December 12, Dr. Andrew T. Still, founder of osteopathy, passes away.

1917 - Mr. Justice Frank Hodgins releases *Report and Supporting Statements on Medical Education in Ontario*. It includes a major review of osteopathic medicine.

1920 - New Brunswick doctors of osteopathy fail in their attempt to obtain separate statutory status but received specific mention in 1920 medical legislation.

1923 - College of Surgeons and Physicians of Ontario supports a regulatory change in the *Medical Act* of 1923 providing for registration of drugless practitioners, such as osteopaths. (The Regulation did not pass.)

1925 - The Ontario provincial government passes the *Drugless Practitioners Act* to regulate osteopathic, chiropractic and other drugless health-care practitioners. The legislation establishes a Board of Regents to govern the practitioners.

1925 - Canadian Osteopathic Association, representing doctors of osteopathy, is formed.

1926 - First regulations under the *Drugless Practitioners Act* in Ontario are published. Under the regulations, osteopaths are entitled to registration if they had graduated from an approved school, were at least 21 years of age and of good character. A grandfather clause covers those who have been practising on January 1, 1926. Doctors are required to pass a Board of Regents' examination.

1929 - Royal College of Physicians and Surgeons of Canada is established under federal law to manage specialist doctors' education.

1933 - Physician/surgeon Dr. F. W. Marlow suggests a chair of osteopathy be established at the University of Toronto.

1934 - Osteopathic and other drugless practitioners sponsor *Bill 86*, which seeks to allow them to use certain occupational titles such as "Doctor", which came under the *Medical Act*. (The Ontario Legislature eventually did not pass it.)

1937 - The Ontario Government passes the *Workmen's Compensation Act* giving doctors of osteopathy the right to treat injured workers.

1937 - Russell C. McCaughan, Executive Secretary of the American Osteopathic Association, urges the Ontario Academy of Osteopaths to set up a board of censors to police its members and to ensure every osteopathic practitioner maintain the highest standards.

1938 - Toronto doctor of osteopathy Hubert J. Pocock declares he cured a patient of arthritis after his case had been given up as "hopeless" by medical men. Calling the patient "Mr. X," Pocock says the patient was bedridden for six months and was told "he would never walk again" prior to his two months of osteopathic treatment.

1940 - Magistrate Jeffs, in a court ruling in Barrie, Ontario, declares a doctor of osteopathy has the right to describe himself after his name, and on his card after his name, as an osteopathic physician. J.E. Wilson is the defendant in a suit brought by the College of Physicians and Surgeons of Ontario.

1941 - Doctor of osteopathy George A. De Jardine, on the recommendation of the Ontario Academy of Osteopathy, is appointed by the Ontario government to the Board of Regents established under the *Drugless Practitioners Act*.

1942 - Doctors of osteopathy in Montreal celebrate the 50th anniversary of the founding of the first osteopathic educational institution in the United States.

1943 - Doctor of osteopathy George A. De Jardine, on behalf of the Canadian Osteopathic Association, presents a brief to the social security committee of the House of Commons, urging the "Dominion Government" to enact legislation regulating the practice of the healing arts in Canada similar to that enacted in the United States, providing "the degrees of doctor of medicine and doctor of osteopathy shall be accorded the same rights and privileges under Government regulation."

1944 - New regulations in Ontario under the *Drugless Practitioners Act* introduce new educational requirements for doctors of osteopathy: Junior matriculation, two years of college, and graduation from a professional osteopathic college with a four-year course.

1944 - Department of National Revenue issues a policy, under the *Income Tax War Act*, that allows payments to osteopaths by patients be counted as medical expenses.

1951 - A motion by Alderman Sparling to permit osteopaths to establish offices in residential areas in Toronto as doctors and dentists can, is turned down at a City Council meeting.

1952 - An Act in Ontario is passed that provides authority for the Lieutenant-Governor in Council to appoint a Board of Directors to govern, separately, osteopaths, chiropractors, masseurs, chiropodists, drugless therapists and physiotherapists. A Board of Osteopathic Practitioners is appointed under the chairmanship of Douglas Firth.

1954 - The College of Family Physicians of Canada is established under federal law to accredit, as a national examining and certifying body, post-graduate family medicine training in Canada's 17 medical schools.

1960 - The Canadian Osteopathic Aid Society announces plans to build a $2-million College of Osteopathy. The college would offer a seven-year course leading to the Doctor of Osteopathy degree.

1965 - Commissioner Gerald Lacroix releases the *Quebec Royal Commission on Chiropraxy and Osteopathy* report.

1966 - Health Minister Allan MacEachen introduces changes to *Canada Health Act* to allow the inclusion of alternate types of treatments such as osteopathy that is to be approved by medical doctors but not performed by them.

1967 - The Castonguay-Nepveu Commission (Commission on Health Care and Social Services) in its report criticizes the power of medicine to control health care. It recommends a new health insurance policy, a new health care network, as well as a new network of social service clinics in Quebec.

1969 - Ontario enters the federal "Medicare" system—Canada's publicly-funded universal health insurance system.

1970 - I.R. Dowie, chair of an Ontario three-person inquiry releases a three-volume report for the Ontario Committee on the Healing Arts, that includes recommendations on osteopathy. Chapter 20 of volume 2 exclusively covers osteopathy.

1970 - Ontario begins, from July 1, providing limited coverage for osteopathic services through the Ontario Health Insurance Plan.

1971 - National health insurance encompasses all provinces.

1972 - "The Hastings Report." Dr. John Hastings and a committee reviews community health centres in Canada and also conducted invitational seminars on physicians services, nursing services and those of allied health personnel.

1981 - Collège d'Études Ostéopathiques in Montreal opens its doors. It is the first in Quebec and Canada to offer a course in non-physician osteopathy.

1982 - The Canadian Foundation for Teaching and Research in Osteopathy, a non-profit body, is founded in Montreal by Philippe Druelle, DO, to promote "traditional "osteopathy" and to help the needy by treating young children with neuromotor dysfunctions.

1989 - Government of Ontario releases *Striking a New Balance: A Blueprint for the Regulation of Ontario's Health Professionals: Recommendations of the Health Professions Legislation Review.*

1992 - Canadian College of Osteopathy (CCO) is established in Toronto.

1993 - The General Osteopathic Council, the United Kingdom's statutory regulator for osteopathy, is established under the *Osteopaths Act* of the same year.

1997 - Canadian Complementary Medicine Association is launched to protect the rights of doctors practising alternative therapies.

1997 - The Ontario Society of Physicians for Complementary Medicine is established to support individual physicians in their practice of complementary medicine.

2000s - The Federation of Medical Regulatory Authorities of Canada develops an agreement which, upon implementation, will establish a national standard for licensure in all jurisdictions.

2001-02 - Montreal-based Collège d'Études Ostéopathiques offers courses in non-physician osteopathy in Vancouver and Halifax.

2002 - Yukon Medical Council, Yukon's medical regulatory authority, is established.

2003 - Holders of the Doctor of Osteopathic Medicine degree issued by an accredited osteopathic medical school in the United States is now recognized by College of Physicians and Surgeons of Ontario, starting in September. The new policy says the degree is equivalent to a degree in medicine as defined in clause (a) of Section 1 of *Ontario Regulation 865/93.*

2003 - L'Association des Ostéopathes du Québec-Canada is launched in Quebec.

2004 - The International Osteopathic Alliance is established in Illinois to unite the osteopathic profession across the globe.

2005 - The International Osteopathic Alliance holds its inaugural conference with 30 international organizations, representing almost a dozen countries.

2008 - The Association of Faculties of Medicine releases a report on *The Future of Medical Education in Canada (FMEC): A Collective Vision for MD Education.*

2009 - The Canadian College of Osteopathy opens a campus in Winnipeg.

2010 - World Health Organization releases report on *Benchmarks for Training in Traditional/Complementary and Alternative Medicine: Benchmarks for Training in Osteopathy.*

2012 - Ostéopathie Québec, Canada's largest association of osteopaths, is established with the merger of the Le Régistre des Ostéopathes du Québec and L'Association des Ostéopathes du Québec.

2013 - In June, registrars of the Canadian provincial and territorial health regulatory authorities sign an agreement in principle to introduce a national standard for licensing medical doctors. The agreement is developed by the Federation of Medical Regulatory Authorities of Canada.

2014 - The Canadian Osteopathic Aid Society announces its intention to apply to the Minister of Industry for leave to surrender its charter pursuant to subsection 32(1) of the *Canada Corporations Act.*

2014 - Quebec-based manual osteopath Ken Montizambert is charged by the Collège des médecins du Québec (Quebec's medical regulatory body) for allegedly practising medicine.

2014 - Offices des professions du Québec announces an initiative, including the creation of committees to investigate the various aspects of osteopathy, that may lead to recommendations regarding a regulatory framework for Quebec manual osteopaths.

Acknowledgements: The Globe and Mail Historical Newspaper Archive; Toronto

Star Historical Newspaper Archive; Ontario. Commission on Medical Education. Report and Supporting Statements on Medical Education in Ontario; and Canada. Royal Commission on Health Services: Study of Chiropractors, Osteopaths and Naturopaths in Canada.

APPENDIX 2—FRIENDLY FIREBRANDS: EARLY CANADIAN OSTEOPATHIC PHYSICIANS

DR. HERST, 1918

"We want osteopathy perpetuated and taught by its followers, not its opponents [medical doctors]."

The Toronto Daily Star,
Feb. 28, 1918.

HUBERT POCOCK, 1937

"The medical profession need have nothing to fear from this new legislation [Workmen's Compensation Act amendment]. It won't jeopardize the medical man because our work is not in his sphere [because we specialize more in displacements, sprains, lifts and kindred ailments]. But I can say that we owe no thanks to the medical profession as a whole for this legislation.

"Had it not been for the efforts of laymen who know the true value of osteopathy, it wouldn't have passed. Individually, I have found medical men top-hole, particularly men with larger practices who do not hesitate to refer cases to us. The College of Physicians and Surgeons has done everything in its power to interfere with the osteopathic profession receiving its due rights."

The Toronto Daily Star,
April 27, 1937.

NORMAN RUTLEDGE, 1938

"Though we are considered unqualified by the medical association [the regulatory and licensing body for medical doctors in Ontario], yet we are not considered so by those who matter most, our patients."

The Globe and Mail,
March 30, 1938.

H. FORRESTER MOORE, 1938

"We [as Canadians] boast of British justice—yet, after a decent training I have to work under a stigma to practice my profession. Our osteopathic differences of opinion in therapeutics as the Ontario law now stands make of me a recognized regular trade union "doctor" or an irregular so-called 'cultist.' I personally have never met a mean medical man in my life, but their group [medical doctors'] attitude reminds me of certain Scribes and Pharisees once so ably condemned".

The Globe and Mail,
April 11, 1938.

JOHN O'CONNOR, 1938

"There is a crying need for examination of the children in schools by osteopathic physicians. Every day osteopaths are asked to handle cases suffering with bad curvature of the spine, which if it had been caught earlier could have saved a lot of trouble. There is work to be done and it is the duty of every osteopath to volunteer his services if we are to develop a fit nation."

The Toronto Daily Star,
March 21, 1938.

ERIC JOHNSTON, 1938

"The fact that osteopathic physicians are not examining children in public schools is as much our sin as anyone else's. It is not up to us to wait until we are asked, but as patriotic Canadians, anxious to see that this country lives up to its heritage of manhood, it is our duty to offer our services and I for one am more than willing to give part of my time."

The Toronto Daily Star,
March 21, 1938.

C.V. HINSPERGER, 1941

"Ontario is the only place in the whole world which has laws governing the practice of osteopathy so ridiculous that osteopathic physicians who are graduates of the same colleges as those in the United States are forbidden to use their degree, Doctor of Osteopathy, or to refer themselves as doctors."

The Globe and Mail,
October 6, 1941.

ERIC B. JOHNSTON, 1942

"There is great support in the United States for the 'Energy for Liberty' program proposed by the Canadian Osteopathic Committee on War Effort."

The Globe and Mail,
May 25, 1942.

J.R. McVITY, 1942

"Canadians will become healthier people by reason of wartime rationing and curtailment of luxuries. Gasoline rationing will force people to walk more, thus reducing 'cardio-vascular disease' especially since overweight and lack of exercise are contributing causes to high blood pressure, heart ailments and other circulatory disorders."

The Globe and Mail,
October 5, 1942.

H.E. MOYER, 1943

"Wrong thinking has much to do with bringing disease. Emotions affect the nerves, the nerves affect the circulation and glands, these in turn affect the chemistry of the blood, and this affects the body tissues. [In other words,] a strong emotion of jealousy tend to cause internal growths, including cancer; hatred affects the heart and blood vessels; fear and worry produces digestive disturbances; and exaggerated sensitivity produces skin eruptions and irritations."

The Globe and Mail,
May 31, 1943.

G.R. CHURCH, 1958

"Graduates of the osteopathic school of medicine, who are recognized in the United States as fully qualified physicians and surgeons, are not so recognized in Canada. Although they take an average of 1,600 more hours of college work than do MD's they are discriminated against by being licensed and regulated under the *Drugless Practitioners Act*, which restricts them from ministering to the ills of the public to the extent that their education and long training warrant."

The Globe and Mail,
October 2, 1958.

VICTOR DE JARDINE, 1972

"MDs corner me and ask me all sorts of questions and they are amazed I've had as thorough an education as they have. They find it hard to comprehend. They come out of medical school believing that if they can't cure it, only God can. They can't understand how a lowly person like an osteopath could possibly do anything."

The Toronto Star,
November 23, 1972.

DOUGLAS FIRTH, 1972

"[Some] doctors find that osteopaths are not quacks or oddballs. They are just as dedicated as the doctors."

The Toronto Star,
November 23, 1972.

DOUGLAS FIRTH, 1981

"Our big concern is the thousands of patients who won't get care, once the 27 osteopaths [remaining in Ontario] die or retire. In Ontario, we're considered a form of quack. They [the provincial medical regulator] have made life so difficult for us we can't refer patients to physicians, we can't use public labs or get x-rays, we can't even send patient to physiotherapists."

The Toronto Star,
May 9, 1981.

About the Authors

ATILY GUNARATNE is an osteopathic manual practitioner currently managing a team of natural health practitioners at the Osteopathic Health Centre in Vaughan, Ontario. His extensive medical training began in his native country of Sri Lanka. Atily moved to Europe and worked as an orthopaedic physiotherapist in the United Kingdom for several years. After arriving in Canada, his fascination with "healing" continued while working in rehabilitation, sports medicine and oncology. In 1977, he had his first introduction to osteopathy when he worked with an orthopaedic surgeon in Europe. Intrigued with this practice and after years of study and practice, he attained his DOMP (Doctorate in Osteopathic Manual Practice) through the Canadian College of Osteopathy in 2000. He combines his passion for "problem solving" with his vast experience, and partners with his team and patients to help the latter achieve a healthier lifestyle. Atily volunteers with Osteopathy Without Borders in Peru, fundraises for the United Way's CN Tower Climb, and mentors osteopathic students. His hobbies include auto racing, photography and gardening.

JOHN YUEN is a freelance journalist in the Greater Toronto Area, specializing in human resources communications and public relations materials for business, non-profit organizations and the public sector. His graduate degree thesis at Carleton University, *Roughing it in the Corporate Bush: Company Editors in Canada and Their Handling of Controversial News*, is an historical study of the politics of Canadian corporate employee news publishing. He has written for several corporate, trade and professional publications in Canada and abroad. He is a former board member (internal communications) of the International Association of Business Communications (IABC/Toronto chapter) and editor of its monthly *IABC Communicator* publication. Prior to freelancing, he was a communications specialist for the Ontario government, the Regional Municipality of Peel, and SONY. He is currently promoting, as a volunteer, career management and community engagement activities at the Human Resources Professionals Association (HRPA) – York Region chapter.

ENDNOTES

[1] https://www.ratemds.com/doctor-ratings/3207080/Dr-Atily-Gunaratne-Mississauga-ON.html Oct. 3, 2014.

[2] http://www.precision-chiropractic.co.uk/blog/2013/05/14/difference-between-a-chiropractor-and-an-osteopath/

[3] Tracey L. Adams, "The Rise and Fall of Osteopathic Medicine in Ontario: 1900-1930s, *Histoire sociale / Social History*, (Ottawa: Les Publications Histoire sociale / Social History Inc., May 2012), p. 51.

[4] See Barbara Clow, *Negotiating Disease: Power and Cancer Care, 1900-1950* (Kingston: McGill-Queen's University Press, 2001) to learn about Canadians' motivation for seeking alternate medical care.

[5] Hans Baer, *Toward an Integrative Medicine: Merging Alternative Therapies with Biomedicine*, (Walnut Creek, CA: Alta Mira Press, 2004), p. 1.

[6] http://translate.google.ca/translate?hl=en&sl=fr&u=http://www.inst-osteopathie.qc.ca/&prev=search Educational Institute of osteopathy Quebec. Nov. 25, 2014.

[7] "Can Treat All Ills Osteopaths Declare: House of Lords . . . Train Most in U.S." (*The Toronto Daily Star,* July 20, 1935), p. 29.

[8] https://www.royal.gov.uk/ThecurrentRoyalFamily/ThePrincessRoyal/Charitiesandpatronages.

[9] "Dean of Windsor Castle says Osteopath Cured Him: Lord Noel-Buxton and Many Others . . . Dispute Raging," (*The Toronto Daily Star*, Dec. 27, 1933), p. 1.

[10] Stephen Gordon, "The Regulation of Complementary Medicine," *Consumer Policy Review*, 7.2 (March 1997): pp. 65-69.

[11] Beverly Smith, "Boileau Returns After Serious Back Surgery: Osteopath Saved her Career, Balancing her Body Alignment , treating her sciatic nerve," (*The Globe and Mail*, April, 19, 2004), p. S8.

[12] Al Strachan, "Clark on the Path to Rejoining Leafs," (*The Globe and Mail*, July 25, 1988), p. C2.

[13] Ontario. Commission on Medical Education. *Report and Supporting Statements on Medical Education in Ontario*, Mr. Justice Hodgins, Commissioner. Vol. 1, (1917), Toronto: A.T. Wilgress, p. 17.

[14] Marilyn Dunlop, "Scorned Here, Osteopaths Can Head Hospitals in U.S.," (*The Globe and Mail*, Nov. 13, 1980), p. A16.

[15] Canada. Royal Commission on Health Services, Donald L. Mills, *Study of Chiropractors, Osteopaths and Naturopaths in Canada* (1966) Ottawa: Queen's Printer,. p. 222.

[16] *Ibid.*, p. 223.

[17] *Ibid.*, p. 225.

[18] *Ibid.*, p. 222.

[19] *Ibid.*

[20] *Ibid.*, p. 224.

[21] Hodgins, op.cit., p. 29.

[22] See Paul Starr, *The Social Transformation of American Medicine: The Rise of a Sovereign Profession and the Making of a Vast Industry.* (New York, NY: Basic Books), 1984.

[23] It is generally acknowledged that physicians and surgeons regulatory groups are not only the most important regulator of the medical professions but enjoy enormous power, prestige and privilege as well as the associated economic benefits. See, for instance, M.S. Staum and D.E. Larsen (eds.), *Doctors, Patients and Society: Power and Authority in Medical Care.* (Waterloo: Wilfred Laurier University Press), 1981, p. 177.

[24] Mills, Study of Chiropractors, *op. cit.*, p. 223.

[25] C. David Naylor, *Private Practice, Public Payment: Canadian Medicare and the Politics of Health Insurance 1911 - 1966*, McGill-Queens University Press, 1986, p. 23.

[26] Adam Scalena, "Defining Quackery: An examination of the Manitoba Medical Profession and the early development of professional unity," *The Journal of the Canadian Chiropractic Association.* September 2006; 50(3): pp. 209-210;

[27] *Ibid.*, p. 209.

[28] Mills, Study of Chiropractors, *op. cit.*, p. 222.

[29] *Ibid.*, p. 222.

[30] Naylor, Private Practice, *op. cit.*, p. 23.

[31] Saskatchewan. Legislative Assembly. Debates and Proceedings. 25th Legislature. 1st Session. (3 May 2005). Regina: Queen's Printer, 2005.

[32] http://esask.uregina.ca/entry/northup_anna_1889-1977.html

[33] Mills, Study of Chiropractors, *op. cit.* p. 224.

[34] Letter to the Editor. (*The Toronto Star.* October 9,1982), p. B2.

[35] Justice Hodgins, Medical Education, *op. cit.*, p. 30

[36] Bill Dampler, "Student Osteopath Joins in Age-Old Medical Battle," (*The Toronto Star,* September 10, 1980), p. A8.

[37] Eugene Forsey, "Osteopathy," Letter to the Editor, (*The Globe and Mail.*, August 6, 1982), p. 6.

[38] Tracey L. Adams, *op. cit.*, p. 51.

[39] Ontario. The Committee on the Healing Arts. *A Legal History of Health Professions in Ontario: A Study for the Committee on the Healing Arts.* Elizabeth MacNab (1970), Toronto: Queen's Printer, p. 139.

[40] W.B. Thistle, "Osteopathy and Chiropractic," *CMA Journal*, (Jan 1, 1926), p. 25.

[41] *Ibid.*

[42] *Naylor, Private Practice, op. cit., p. 23.*

[43] J.W.S. MCCullough, "The Medical Profession of Ontario Versus Irregular Practitioners," *The Public Health Journal* 6, 12, (December 1915), p. 617. Quoting Abraham Flexner, *Carnegie Foundation Bulletin Number Four, 1910.*

[44] October 9, 1982.

[45] October 9, 1982.

[46] August 17, 1974.

[47] Justice Hodgins, Medical Education, *op. cit.*, p. 28.

[48] Elizabeth MacNab, *op. cit.*, p. 139.

[49] "Osteopaths Put Under Thumb of Medical College," *(The Toronto Daily Star*, April 4, 1912), p. 3.

[50] Naylor, Private Practice, *op. cit.*, p. 23.

[51] Justice Hodgins, Medical Education, *op. cit.*, p. 3.

[52] *Ibid.*, p. 29.

[53] *Ibid.*, p. 19.

[54] http://www.lawofcanada.net/statutes/r-s-o-1990-c-d-18/1

[55] Ontario. Committee on the Healing Arts., *Report of the Committee on the Healing Arts.* I.R. Dowie, (1970), Toronto: Queen's Printer, Vol. 1, p. 78.

[56] www.publications.gov.sk.ca/redirect.cfm?p=32792&i=39792

[57] *The Globe and Mail*, May 18, 1937, p. 7.

[58] *The Toronto Daily Star*, April 27, 1937, p. 21.

[59] "Committee Hears Osteopaths' Case: Bill Sent on by Legislature Last Year Is Under Consideration," *The Globe*, January 25, 1934, p. 5.

[60] "Queen's Park Kills Bill of Osteopaths: Committee Named to Devise Scheme for Ensuring Proper Status," *(The Toronto Daily Star*, April 11, 1933), p. 2.

[61] "Osteopaths Charge MD's Made Sketchy Inquiries: Spent Less Than Three Hours in Leading College, They Claim," *The Toronto Daily Star*, March 8, 1934, p. 1.

[62] J.R.G. McVity Letter to the Editor *(The Globe and Mail*, Oct. 28, 1942).

[63] G.A. DeJardene, Letter to Editor, *(The Globe and Mail*, June 16, 1943).

[64] "Fitness Needs for War Told to Osteopaths: Industrial . . . Should be Modernized, Convention is Advised," *(The Globe and Mail*, May 25, 1942), p. 5.

[65] Members of the first board were: Douglas Firth representing the Ontario Osteopathic Association (chair); J.R.F McVity (vice-chair); D.G.A Campbell (secretary/treasurer);. Ray Linnen of Ottawa (member); Norman Burbidge of Guelph (member); and a ministry of health representative.

[66] "Ontario Osteopaths Win battle, are Granted Self rule," (*The Toronto Daily Star*, November 6, 1952), p. 1.

[67] *Ibid.*, p. 60.

[68] Ontario. Committee on the Healing Arts. Ian R. Dowie. *Report of the Healing Arts Committee*, Vol. 1, p. vii.

[69] Ibid. Vol. 2, p. 348.

[70] : Eighteenth-century economist Adam Smith had called for free market forces to prevail, and similar thoughts were expressed by those after him such as Murray N. Rothbard and Friedrich A Hayek in the 1970s.

[71] Marilyn Dunlop, "Osteopaths Fear their Healing Art Could Disappear," (*The Toronto Star*, Nov. 23, 1972), p. 8.

[72] *Ibid.*, p. 8.

[73] Editorial. (*The Toronto Star*. May 31, 1974).

[74] "Canada's Osteopaths Deserve a Better Deal," (*The Toronto Star*, June 3, 1970).

[75] Editorial. "Osteopathy Too Valuable to be Lost," (*The Toronto Star*, Aug. 17, 1974).

[76] Michael Tutton, "A return to a hands-on approach to care," (*The Globe and Mail*, September 8, 2011), p. L6.

[77] "Osteopathists to have bill: Seek legislation to enable them to treat what patients they see fit," *The Toronto Daily Star*, December 5, 1906, p. 8.

[78] De Jardine, who in 1972 was the president of the Ontario Osteopathic Association, told the media, "After practising nothing but manipulation for 20 years, Ontario osteopaths would be too rusty to give full [medical] care [they were trained to provide in the U.S. like medical doctors.], according to Marilyn Dunlop "Osteopaths Fear Their Healing Art Could Disappear" (*The Toronto Star*, Nov. 23, 1972), p. 8.

[79] Marilyn Dunlop, *ibid.*, p.8.

[80] Ontario. Legislative Assembly. *Debates and Proceedings*. 34th Parliament. 1st Session. (26 January 1989). Toronto: Hansard Transcripts, 1989.

[81] Patricia O'Reilly, *Health Care Practitioners: An Ontario Case Study in Policy Making*, (Toronto: University of Toronto Press, 2000), p. 38.

[82] Ernie Stapleton & Allen Shiffman, " 'Fringe' healers seek more status" (*The Toronto Star*, October 20, 1983), p. A25.

[83] Stapleton & Shiffman, Ibid.

[84] Ann Silverslides, "Ontario adds Midwives to professional groups regulated by province," (*The Toronto Star*, April 4, 1986), p. A17.

[85] In April 2015, there were 28 self-regulated health professions in Ontario: Audiology and Speech-Language Pathology, Chiropody, Chiropractic, Dental Hygiene, Dental Technology, Dentistry, Denturism, Dietetics, Transitional Council of Homeopathy, Transitional Council of Kinesiology, Massage Therapy, Medical Laboratory Technology, Medical Radiation Technology, Medicine, Midwifery, Transitional Council of Naturopathy, Nursing, Occupational Therapy, Opticianry, Optometry, Pharmacy, Physiotherapy, Psychology, Transitional Council of Psychotherapy, Registered Practical Nursing, Respiratory Therapy, Transitional Council of Traditional Chinese Medicine and Acupuncturists, and Veterinary Medicine.

[86] http://www.cpso.on.ca/Policies-Publications/Policy/Doctors-of-Osteopathic-Medicine, December 2014.

[87] Chapter 7 of the AIT (Agreement on Internal Trade) aims to provide unrestricted mobility between provinces and the territories for workers. According to Industry Canada, "modern internal trade rules [like the AIT) should allow you [as workers] to move freely across domestic borders to pursue career opportunities and find fulfilling jobs anywhere in Canada.) http://www.ic.gc.ca/eic/site/081.nsf/eng/00002.html.

[88] Mark Brownlee, "Doctors Still Face Issues Moving Between Provinces," (*The Globe and Mail*). http://www.theglobeandmail.com/life/health-and-fitness/doctors-still-face-issues-moving-between-provinces/article588975/

[89] *Ibid.*

[90] http://www.osteopathic.ca/

[91] Letter to the Editor. David Fiddler & James Church "Misuse of *Osteopathic* in Non-Physician Titles a Setback for Profession in Canada." *The DO*, American Osteopathic Association, Feb. 17, 2011. http://thedo.osteopathic.org/2011/02/misuse-of-osteopathic-in-nonphysician-titles-a-setback-for-profession-in-canada/

[92] Ted Finlay, "Traditional osteopathy": An oxymoron? Letter to the Editor, *JAOA* (September 2000), p. 545.

[93] David Fiddler and James Church, *op. cit.* Note: The OIA has also admitted other Canadian non-physician groups as "partner members," such as Ostéopathie Québec, the Ontario Association of Osteopathic Manual Practitioners, and the British Columbia–based Society for the Promotion of Manual Practice Osteopathy (SPMPO).

[94] Carolyn Schierhorn, "Somatic, semantic distinctions: DOs try to come to terms with manual therapists," *The DO* (Jan. 7, 2011).

[95] Its 2015 international officers are: Christine Marechal and Christie Lythgoe of Calgary; Andrew Bi and Lynda Simpson of Toronto; Nick Church of Victoria; Chris Jacob, Dennis Fiddler and Iain Jeffery of Whitby, Lindsay, and Peterborough, Ontario, respectively; Niraj Patel of the Greater Toronto Area; and Lauren McLaughlin of Halifax. They are attending one of the 30 American Osteopathic Association-recognized colleges of osteopathic medicine in the U.S.: The colleges have altogether 40 locations for instructing their students, according to Nicole Grady, in a February 25, 2015. e-mail, from the American Osteopathic Association.

[96] Gail Abernethy, Personal Interview, January 25, 2015.

[97] http://wp.oialliance.org/wp-content/uploads/2013/07/canada_osteopathy.pdf Dec. 20, 2014.

[98] *Dr. Sicotte passed away as this book was being edited.

[99] http://wp.oialliance.org/wp-content/uploads/2013/06/OAO-Partner-Profile-Summary-2015.pdf

[100] Nadeem Esmail, "Complementary and Alternative Medicine in Canada: Trends in Use and Public Attitudes, 1997–2006," *Public Policy Sources* 87 (May 2007):. pp. 22, 52.

[101] https://professions-Québec.org/en/the-professional-system/

[102] Stéphan Boivin, Office des professions du Québec, e-mail, April 12, 2015.

[103] Boivin, *ibid.*

[104] Personal Interview Chantale Bertrand, November 5, 2014.

[105] E-mail. Jean Guy Sicotte, MD DO (Q.), Oct. 4, 2007.

[106] http://www.college-osteopathes.org/ Google translation from French to English.

[107] http://www.osteopathie-canada.ca/en/page/general-profile

[108] http://translate.google.ca/translate?hl=en&sl=fr&u=http://www.inst-osteopathie.qc.ca/&prev=search

[109] http://translate.google.ca/translate?hl=en&sl=fr&u=http://www.aomtl.ca/&prev=search

[110] http://www.aomtl.ca/?gclid=CL7Kks3gvsMCFZE1aQodeCMAPw

[111] http://www.academiesutherland.com/en/about/about03.php

[112] Académie Sutherland d'Ostéopathie du Québec class handout. N.p.

[113] http://www.coqm.qc.ca/

[114] http://www.epoqosteopathie.com/

[115] http://www.cmq.org/en/ObtenirPermis/DiplomesCanadaUS.aspx Jan. 15, 2014

[116] http://montreal.ctvnews.ca/controversial-pointe-claire-osteopath-ordered-to-stop-medical-treatments-1.1924395 January 15, 2015.

[117] *Ibid.*

[118] http://www.cpso.on.ca/CPSO/media/uploadedfiles/policies/policies/policyitems/Doctors-Osteopathic-Medicine.PDF?ext=.pdf

[119] http://www.greatwestlife.com/001/Home/Individual_Products/Insurance/Health_Dental_Insurance/EnhancedHealthcare-PlanDirect/Plan_Designs/Detailed_Coverage_Information/index.htm

[120] Kathryn Clarke, CPSO. E-mail. Sept. 15, 2014.

[121] http://www.payscale.com/research/CA/Job=Physician_%2f_Doctor%2c_General_Practice/Salary. The terms "Physician / Doctor, General Practice Salary" in the search function were used.

[122] The History Of Naturopathic Medicine: A Canadian Perspective, 2009, Toronto: McArthur & Co. p.100.

[123] Tracey L. Adams, *op. cit.,* p. 51.

[124] http://www.cmaj.ca/content/160/6/877.full.pdf

[125] http://www.cpso.on.ca/policies-publications/policy/complementary-alternative-medicine Nov. 5, 2014

[126] Dundas Bradley, Personal Interview, October 28, 2014.

[127] Chantal Roy, Personal Interview, October 5, 2015.

[128] *Osteopathy Research and Practice,* 1910, p.7

[129] E-mail, Nov. 30, 2014.

[130] http://www.osteopathycentre.ca/aboutus.html Dec. 10, 2014

[131] Personal Interview, Dec. 14, 2014

[132] http://torontoosteopathy.com/ Dec. 17, 2014

[133] ttp://pathstovitality.com/blog/ Dec. 18, 2014

[134] Harvard Gazette "Admissions, beyond a single test" http://news.harvard.edu/gazette/story/2013/03/admissions-beyond-a-single-test/ Nov 20, 2014.

[135] The responses from the leaders of Ontario's manual osteopathic schools and groups can be a treasure trove of data for public policy makers and the public. Unfortunately, several associations and schools did not respond to multiple requests from the authors of this book, requesting comment on these questions.

[136] http://wp.oialliance.org/wp-content/uploads/2013/07/canada_osteopathy.pdf.

[137] Under an agreement signed between one of the book authors and the Canadian Academy of Osteopathy, it is not possible to describe the school's information. Please visit its website.

[138] http://www.osteopathiecollege.com/new/program_five_years_study.php.

[139] http://www.numss.com/

[140] http://www.osteopathycollege.com/uploads/6/0/9/8/6098453/oso_catalogue-2014-15_-_new_footer.pdf page 9. Nov. 22, 2014

[141] http://www.osteopathycollege.com/uploads/6/0/9/8/6098453/osteopathy_student_handbook_-_2013-14.pdf.

[142] http://www.clinicalosteopathy.com/college.html Nov. 23, 2014.

[143] http://www.o-c-o.org/ Nov. 22, 2014

[144] http://lcocanada.com/product/osteopathy-facial-esthetics/

[145] Kelly Eby, director of communications, E-mail, CPSA, dated Aug. 26, 2014.

[146] Shan Rupnarain, Assistant Executive Director, Public Affairs, E-mail, Aug. 26, 2014.

[147] http://osteopathyalberta.com.

[148] http://www.osteopathy.ca/associations, Nov. 30, 2014.

[149] *Ibid.*

[150] U.S.-trained doctors of osteopathic medicine who emigrated to Alberta before and after 1905 when the province became part of Canada, first got regulated in 2011. Under an amendment to the 1906 *Health Professions Act* that took effect in December 20 of that year, the Council of the College of Physicians and Surgeons of Alberta admitted the osteopaths to the medical registry once they tendered a valid certificate from the Registrar of the University of Alberta indicating they were "duly qualified." The examination of candidates for admission to practice, the Council agreed, was to be carried out by the university. For more information, please consult the website:: http://archive.org/stream/albertamedicalre1911coll/albertamedicalre1911coll_djvu .txt

The examinations, under the auspices of the University of Alberta, focused on anatomy, physiology, chemistry, toxicology, pathology, bacteriology, histology, neurology, physical diagnosis, obstetrics, gynecology, surgery, hygiene, medical jurisprudence, and principles and practice of osteopathy.

The osteopathic physicians' status was short-lived, however. In 1948, they were put under the umbrella of the 1948 *Drugless Practitioners Act* in the province. Like

Ontario's osteopathic doctors, they were not allowed to use the title "Doctor," prohibited from performing normal medical doctor duties for which they were qualified in the U.S., and therefore only practised osteopathic manipulative medicine.

While the DOs were flourishing in the U.S.—with most jurisdictions in the 1950s granting them full practice rights—Alberta's handful of DOs did not do so well.

The attitude of the College of Physicians and Surgeons of Alberta (CPSA) was one of concern that "DOs coming in who are less qualified than allopaths (medical

doctors)," according to Charlotte Gray. "Osteopathy: Is there a Place in Canadian Medicine," *CMA Journal*, July 1, 1981, p.111.

But in the 1970s, as a result of increasing public demand for osteopaths' skills, pressure from osteopaths across the country and support from ordinary Canadians who benefited from osteopathic treatments, the tide turned, Gray noted. The CPSA acknowledged it was behind the times. Said the CPSA's Dr. Le Riche, commenting on the lack of policy direction on osteopathy from the Canadian Medical Association`s Council on Medical Education: "It's a conundrum that the provinces have not, at the moment, come to grips with."

In April 1972,.in commissioning the Special Legislative Committee on Professions and Occupations, the Alberta government chose to include health disciplines in the inquiry's mandate. A policy paper was issued in 1978—and revised six years later—a follow-up on the findings of the committee report and stipulated that "all persons practising a regulated profession or occupation must be licensed and the field of practice must be clearly described, noted Dr. J.P. Boase. *Shifting Sands: Government-*

Group Relationships in the Health Care Sector. 1994. McGill-Queens University Press, p. 78

Bill 84 was introduced in October 1980 and passed as the *Health Occupations Act*. It sought to establish a mechanism by which the government can respond in a timely fashion to the demands of unregulated health professions—such as osteopathy—for regulation. The Health Occupations Board was one of the outcomes. The board was mandated to advise the government on regulating these occupations. By 1983, five occupations—that did not include osteopathy—were designated. *The Health Occupations Act* morphed and became *the Health Disciplines Act*. Boase noted. With the change in name of the legislation, the Health Occupations Board became the Health Disciplines Board.

Alberta's osteopathic manual practitioners who are familiar with the medical history of the province revel in the fact that their osteopathic manipulation techniques were earlier championed by an Albertan medical doctor long ago. Dr. W.B. Parsons, of the Town of Sylvan Lake, a well-known tourist area, had many times urged his peers to refer their patients to the few osteopathic physicians in the province before and during 1980s. "[I]n view of the improved status of the osteopaths, maybe the physician who doesn't manipulate should refer cases to them," he wrote.

In a letter to the editor of the journal of the Canadian Medical Association, the physician lauded manual manipulation as a pain reliever and urged it become "part of the physician's 'armamentarium.' " Parsons said he spent his "lifetime" trying to

persuade the medical profession, through articles, letters and demonstration, of the value of manipulation and to adopt its use. (see W.B. Parsons, "Osteopathy," Letter to the Editor, *CMA Journal* 126, (Feb. 1, 1982), p. 231.)

[151] http://nmoc.ca/

[152] Susan Prins. College of Physicians and Surgeons of British Columbia. E-mail. Aug. 29, 2014.

[153] *COMLEX (Comprehensive Osteopathic Medical Licensing Examination); USMLE (The United States Medical Licensing Examination); FLEX (Federation Licensing Examination); NBME (National Board of Medical Examiners).

[154] Prins, e-mail, *op.cit.*

[155] Personal Interview with Julie Brown, Nov. 27, 2014

[156] http://cpsm.mb.ca/registration.

[157] E-mail, dated Aug. 26, 2014.

[158] http://www.canadianbiologics.com/index.html.

[159] Personal Interview with Dr. Paul Conyette, Sept.9, 2014.

[160] http://www.canadianbiologics.com/index.html.

[161] http://www.osteopathy.ca/associations.

[162] www.osteopathy.ca Retrieved Sept. 7, 2014.

[163] http://www.princeton.edu/~achaney/tmve/wiki100k/docs/Common_law.html

[164] www.osteopathy.ca

[165] Saint John, New Brunswick's largest city and the capital, was, according to Emmons Rutledge Booth writing in 1905, the location where Canada's first osteopath, established a practice. Dr. H.L. Spangler, the author claimed, was the first osteopath to introduce osteopathy into the country, (See E.R. Booth, *History of Osteopathy and Twentieth Century Medical Practice*. (Cincinnati: Jennings and Graham, 1905) p.70.)) Booth also wrote that the number of practitioners "at St. Johns [sic] ' grew' in favor till there are now [1905] about twenty-five practising in the most important centers of population in the dominion." Source: *Ibid.*

[166] E-mail. Dated Aug. 26, 2014.

[167] http://nslegislature.ca/index.php/proceedings/hansard/C81/house_11may06/#HPage1905

[168] *Ibid.*

[169] W.M. Lowe. Letter. College of Physicians and Surgeons of Nova Scotia, September 25, 2014.

[170] During the 1970s, attempts were made to rationalize its legislation in this area. In 1972 and 1976, for example, government-sponsored inquiries by the Nova Scotia Council of Health and the Nova Scotia Committee on Health Professions Licensing respectively, made recommendations toward that end. Political scientist Dr. J.P. Boase observer noted that there were "few concrete results." Please see, *Shifting Sands: Government-Group Relationships in the Health Care Sector*. 1994. McGill-Queens University Press, p. 82.

[171] http://www.novascotiaosteopaths.ca/wp/osteopathy-in-canada/and http://www.osteopathy.ca/associations/

[172] College of Nurses of Nova Scotia. *Transitioning to Professional Practice: A Resource for Recent Graduates Planning to Register with the College of Registered Nurses of Nova Scotia*, (Halifax: The College of Registered Nurse of Nova Scotia), 2013, p. 5.

[173] http://www.gov.nu.ca/health/information/about-us. Additional information is available on: http://en.wikipedia.org/wiki/Inuit_Qaujimajatuqangit

[174] http://www.nunavut-physicians.gov.nu.ca/index.shtml

[175] http://www.gov.nu.ca/health/information/about-us

[176] Melissa Macdonald. E-mail, Aug. 29, 2014.

[177] http://cpspei.ca/wp-content/uploads/2012/04/REGULATIONS-FOR-PEI-Approved-Changes-as-of-May-12014.pdf

[178] http://www.gov.pe.ca/index.php3/newsroom/index.php3?number=news&newsnumber=8550&dept=&lang=E

[179] http://www.health.gov.sk.ca/professional-associations

[180] http://www.cps.sk.ca/Documents/Legislation/Legislation/Regulatory%20Bylaws%20-%20April%202015.pdf

[181]. Bryan Salte, Q.C. Associate Registrar, Saskatchewan College of Physicians and Surgeons, E-mail. March 11, 2015.

[182] The Saskatchewan Society of Osteopathic Physicians represented osteopathic physicians before it became defunct with the repeal of the *Osteopathic Practice Repeal Act* in 2005.

For about 60 years, prior to 2005, however, Saskatchewan-based osteopathic medicine doctors, or , who graduated from recognized U.S. osteopathic colleges ordered X-rays, were allowed to write prescriptions and performed surgery just like medical doctors. Those professional arrangements, including the Society and title and scope of practice protection for doctors of osteopathy, ended at midnight on Thursday, May 26, 2005 with *The Osteopathic Practice Repeal Act,* passed by the New Democratic (NDP) government of Lorne A. Calvert.

Ironically, the original legislation, *The Osteopathic Practice Act* of 1944, was enacted by a CCF, or Co-operative Commonwealth Federation, government (the CCF being the predecessor political party to the New Democrats).

The 1944 legislation conferred doctors of osteopathic medicine with full professional status. It created a Board of Osteopathic Physicians of three to five persons. It also made bylaws for registering osteopathic physicians as members, and admitting osteopathic physicians to practise. The legislation stated members must have attended a recognized osteopathic training institution that provided a resident course of four school or college periods of nine months each or more, and had, as a

prerequisite of entrance, two years of university and pre-osteopathic education including courses in English, physics, chemistry and biology, that is recognized at an approved osteopathic college by the American Osteopathic Association.

The Board was also empowered to make membership open to any person who has been engaged in the actual practice of osteopathy for a period of ten years or more immediately prior to the first day of April, 1944, and who furnished evidence of qualifications and moral character satisfactory to it. For additional information, please see ttp://www.qp.gov.sk.ca/documents/English/Statutes/Repealed/O7.pdf

Prior to 1944, osteopathic doctors, along with chiropractors had been caught in a struggle with medical doctors who objected to other health care groups getting regulatory status. According to researcher Sharon Baldwin, this struggle "came to a head" in 1917, although an Act to regulate the practice of osteopathy was passed in 1913. On that fateful year, the government passed *The Drugless Practitioners Act,* or DPA, covering both osteopathic doctors and chiropractors. The new law protected osteopaths and chiropractors from prosecution by defining their methods outside the practice of medicine or surgery. But the inter-professional conflicts continued even after the DPA was proclaimed. (Source: Sharon Baldwin, *Self-interest and the Public Interest: Professional regulation in Saskatchewan, 1905-1948.*, MA Thesis, University of Regina. June 1998.)

Due to the constant bickering between the two professions in the 1940s, the people of Saskatchewan developed a negative view of these professions. Baldwin described the reputation of the groups then as being "devalued".

The Select Standing Committee on Law Amendments was appointed in 1946 by the government. The CCF government charged the committee to "investigate professional associations by studying the Acts, bylaws and regulations," and focus on membership qualifications, and exams and appeal provisions for members who had to be disciplined.

As a result of the investigations, the committee proposed a "Professional Associations Act" to create 19 "special administration boards" to oversee the professions. It also proposed the University of Saskatchewan manage the examinations for the professions. The bill, however, died after a furor from the media, in particular, the *Financial Post*, the public and the federal government.

[183] Personal Interview. Nov. 4, 2014.

[184] http://www.yukonmedicalcouncil.ca/ Oct.7, 2014.

[185] http://www.yukonmedicalcouncil.ca/physician_licensing.html Oct.7, 2014.

[186]Karen Lincoln, Medical Council Coordinator, Professional Licensing & Regulatory Affairs, E-mail. August 28, 2014.

[187] Sohrab Khoshbin, Personal Interview, October 30, 2014

[188] Gail Abernethy, Personal Interview, January 25, 2015

[189] Paul Pross, Personal Interview, February 11, 2015.

[190] Jillian Kohler, Personal Interview, February 12, 2015.

[191] http://ofop.ca/ Jan. 25, 2015

[192] http://www.ontarioosteopathyboard.org/ Jan. 25, 2015

[193] http://osteopathyontario.org/our-association/ Jan. 25, 2015.

[194]http://www.internationalosteopathicassociation.org/about_ioa.html. Jan. 25, 2015.

[195] The school representatives said: (1) both authors had to be present at the interview [the book authors viewed this as an unreasonable use of their time and resources] and (2) the school insisted they must approve what is written about it in the book [the book authors interpreted this as an unwarranted restriction on journalistic freedom].

[196] A major illustration of Prof. O'Reilly's published work on the politics of Ontario's health professions can be found in Patricia O'Reilly, *Health Care Practitioners: An Ontario Case Study in Policy Making* (Toronto: University of Toronto Press, 2000).

[197] Patricia O'Reilly, e-mail, November 25, 2014.

[198] *Evidence and Healthy Public Policy: Insights from Health and Political Sciences. Proceedings of Workshop,* Ottawa, March 5, 2007, ed. Patrick Farfard. Ottawa: National Collaborating Centre for Healthy Public Policy and Institut national de santé publique, May 2008, p. 14. http://www.cprn.org/documents/50036_EN.pdf

[199] We borrow the phrase "enabling environment" from the United Nations Sustainable Development literature, and narrowed its meaning here to suggest that changes of a cooperative nature will help health-care practitioner advocacy groups get more mileage in their quest for getting attention from the regulatory authorities.

[200] Joan P. Boase, "Regulation and the Paramedical Professions: An Interest Group Study," *Canadian Public Administration* 25, 3, (September 1982): p. 332.

[201] Elizabeth Leach, Personal Interview, September 12, 2014.

[202] Hugh.M. Cuthbertson, Carl J. Denbow & Guido H. Stempel III, "David and Goliath Co-exist: The Story of Osteopathic Public Relations," *Political, and Economic Contexts in Public Relations: Theory and Cases* (London: Routledge Communication Series, 1993), pp. 227 - 269.

[203] https://bojinkab.wordpress.com/2010/01/14/hugh-culbertson-weighs-in/

[204] http://osteopathichistory.com/pdfs/OsteopathyUndivided.pdf March 4, 2015.

[205] Personal Interview. March 8, 2015.

INDEX

CPSIA information can be obtained at www.ICGtesting.com
Printed in the USA
LVOW07s0254271015

459849LV00009B/48/P